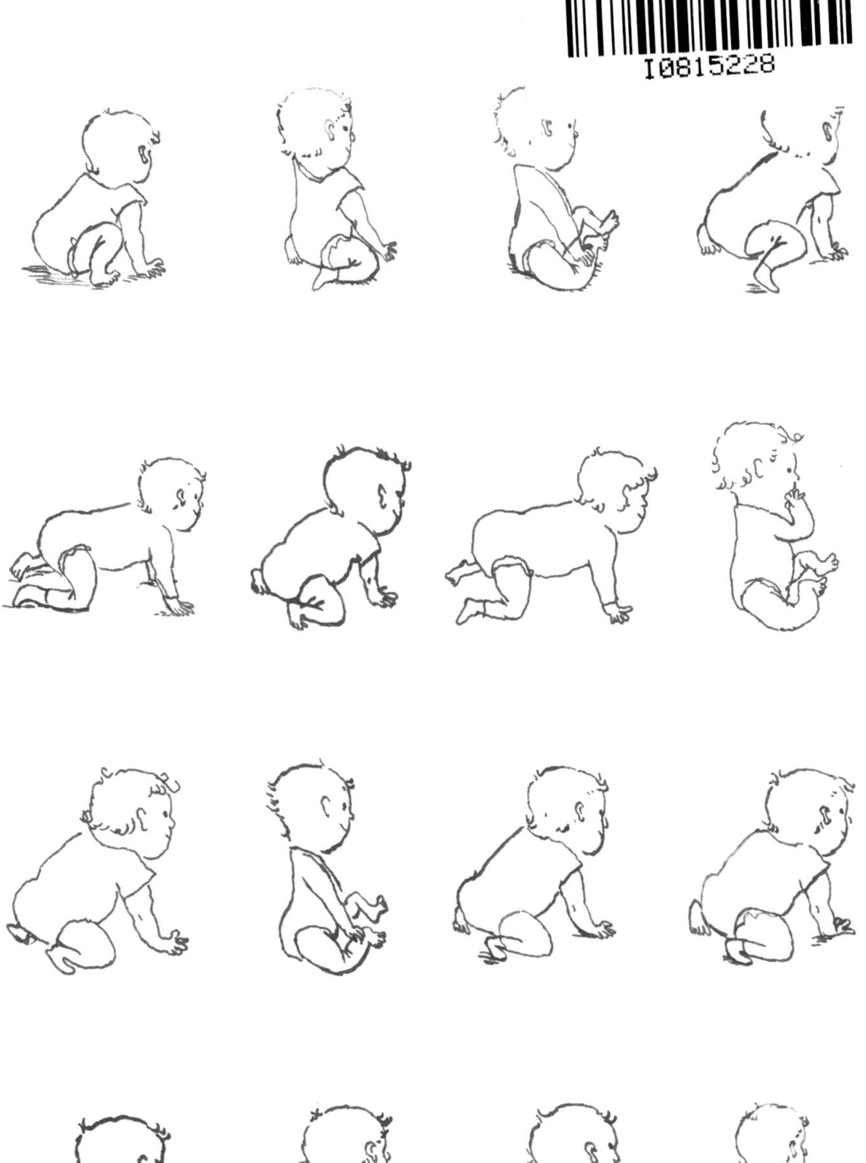
I0815228

The Republic of Parenthood

Also by Rhiannon Lucy Cosslett:

Fiction
The Tyranny of Lost Things
Female, Nude

Non-fiction
The Vagenda (co-author with Holly Baxter)
The Year of the Cat

Also by Pia Bramley:
Pandemic Baby

The Republic of Parenthood

On Bringing Up Babies

Rhiannon Lucy Cosslett

Illustrated by Pia Bramley

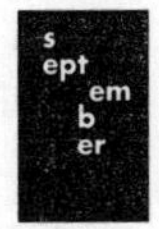

First published in the United Kingdom by September Publishing in 2025

September Publishing, an imprint of Duckworth Books Ltd
1 Golden Court, Richmond, TW9 1EU, United Kingdom
www.duckworthbooks.co.uk

Copyright © Rhiannon Lucy Cosslett, 2025
Illustrations copyright © Pia Bramley, 2025

All rights reserved. No part of this publication may be reproduced, stored in a retrieval system, or transmitted, in any form or by any means electronic, mechanical, photocopying, recording or otherwise, without the prior permission of the publisher.

The right of Rhiannon Lucy Cosslett to be identified as the Author of this Work has been asserted by her in accordance with the Copyright, Designs and Patents Act 1988.

A catalogue record for this book is available from the British Library

Lines on p. 2 from 'The Republic of Motherhood' by Liz Berry.

Design and typesetting by Danny Lyle

Printed and bound in Great Britain by CPI Books

The authorised representative in the EEA is Easy Access System Europe, Mustamäe tee 50, 10621 Tallinn, Estonia.

Hardback ISBN: 9780715655856
eISBN: 9780715655863

For our little Bug

Contents

Introduction

'Nothing prepares you.'

That's what people say about parenthood, and I'm afraid that it is true. If you have picked up this book in the hope that it might act as a guide – either for you as a parent-to-be or for a loved one embarking on this journey – please don't put it down just yet. Hear me out!

There are, of course, things that you can do to get ready for the arrival of a baby in your life. You can go to National Childbirth Trust (NCT) classes (or one of the other courses, such as Bump & Baby which are, apparently, a tad more positive about epidurals). You can decorate a nursery, which may be used mostly as a very beautiful storage cupboard if your baby insists on sleeping next to you. You can pack your hospital bag; actually, this is something I highly recommend that you do, lest your waters go early and explosively, and you and your partner end up running around the flat putting random shit in a bag as the taxi to the hospital pulls up outside, only for you to realise twenty-four hours later, when you've *just given birth to an actual baby*, that you forgot to pack a nightie, meaning you have to ask your husband to bring you one, only for him to turn up with a suitcase of completely unsuitable silky negligees, meaning you eventually have to buy one off Amazon. Just speaking from experience.

In fact, if you'd like to take this moment to pack your hospital bag now, please do, I'll still be here when you get back.

So yes, there are things you can do. Most helpfully of all, you can read books and articles about other people's experience, as research. Like many, many parents before me, I embarked upon this endeavour with great enthusiasm. Surely, I assumed, if I read widely and deeply enough, motherhood will not be *that* much of a shock. Yet, despite the fact that billions of human beings have become parents, far fewer of us have written about it, especially women. Owing to the twin challenges of patriarchy and death in childbirth, the literature of motherhood remains in its, well, infancy. Some of the books I read were truly terrible; for me, personally, there is a special place in hell for *The Little Book of Self-Care for New Mums*. A friend, meanwhile, said she threw *The Wonder Weeks* straight in the recycling. Each parent has their own *bêtes noires*. But most were excellent, and all of them taught me something, even if I disagreed with them. I have referred to and been in conversation with many of these authors throughout my column series and therefore this book. But did they prepare me? No. Because nothing bloody does.

Becoming a parent is one of the most significant things that can ever happen to a person, and it is never not going to be a shock. Even the most brilliant, insightful writer in the world will struggle to convey the sheer, miraculous, terrifying, all-consuming viscerality of parenthood. Having a child is like being hit by a tsunami. Not a bad one, necessarily. The tsunami is made of love, a love that at times feels like it borders on insanity, or grief, or the high you get from MDMA. The tsunami is also made of shit, though. Shit and milk, and this substance called lochia, which hardly anyone knows about until it starts coming out of them. If you want to Google lochia, I am also happy to wait.

As I wrote at the time, motherhood feels as though you have woken up in Oz and everything's in Technicolor. But also, you've been crushed by a house.

It is this mix of complicated, amplified feelings that I think is lacking from so much writing about parenthood. Just as people will tell you that the days are long and the years are short (and people will tell you this a lot), you'll discover that while the highs may be higher than any you've felt before, my God, the lows can be very low. The nights, meanwhile, are strange indeed. Some nights may feel agonisingly lonely; on others you may feel you're losing your grip on reality. On these nights, you might feel as though you can't carry on, and have to try to remind yourself that it is well documented that those horrendous hours right before the sun comes up feel the worst, psychologically.

Yet, there will be other nights with your baby where it feels as though the two of you are floating together on a starlit sea, warm and cosy and safe together on a raft made of duvet. On these nights, you need nothing beyond each other and the moon that guides you, and these sensations of closeness, safety and kinship seem the greatest truths you've ever known.

Why is this nuance so often missing from writing about parenthood? In the years since pitching the column to my editors at the *Guardian*, I have frequently pondered this question. When it comes to parenthood – and particularly motherhood – there is always a prevailing wind. For most of human history, motherhood was essentially a cult of positivity. A few mere decades ago, in large part thanks to feminism, came a warts-and-all, truth-telling backlash, when many courageous women writers faced huge stigma to speak honestly about their experiences. As I write this, the wind has changed; the charge against modern mothers seems to be that we are too negative, and wouldn't it be nice if people talked more about the lovely things about motherhood? No doubt, the wind will change several times again between me writing this introduction and this book hitting the shelves.

In writing about my own experience of parenthood, I have been less interested in questions of positivity and negativity than I am in the idea of truth. Everyone's experience of parenthood – or not-parenthood, if that is what you choose, or if it chooses you – is different. Whether a writer is beaming with joy at her baby's first smiles or weeping while covered in sick, these are both valid experiences. Where the difficulty occurs, though, is *when* the writing happens. So much of parenthood is written in retrospect that it is impossible to really feel the truth of the experience, particularly when it comes to those early, delirious nights.

Try asking your own parents, grandparents, or friends about those first years, and most will admit to having huge gaps in their memories; many will also suffer from a kind of selective amnesia, where they have omitted the parts that are less likely to cover them in glory. And I get it. Already, the way I felt while writing those early columns seems oddly remote and intangible. Had I not written about those days and weeks and months, I very much doubt I would be able to reconstruct them from memory. Certainly, if you tasked me to write about breastfeeding now, I'd probably come back with a fairly upbeat piece, despite the agonising pain and desperate sadness I felt when it just wasn't working, when all I wanted in the world was to be able to feed my tiny, pre-term baby. Capturing that rawness was part of my motivation for writing the column in the first place. I wanted it to be not only an examination of the political, philosophical and cultural context of modern parenthood, but also a diaristic account of this major life transition, written in real time.

At the time, I did not realise how ambitious this was because, as I said, nothing prepares you. 'I'll do a few columns in advance and then take a month off,' I thought blithely, 'and then I'll crack on with it.' I had not bargained on my baby coming early, nor had I realised how all-consuming those early days would be. I did not know that the parents of pre-term infants can experience far higher levels of stress than the parents of full-term infants in the first year. If I had, maybe I never would have embarked upon *The Republic of Parenthood* in the first place. As it was, I started making notes before we'd even left the hospital. I had just been through this life-changing, not to mention at times quite frightening, birth, and there was so much that I found myself wanting to say. I suppose that's the writer in me.

Occasionally, people would come up to me and would tell me that they didn't understand how I was doing it. I always felt a little embarrassed when they said this, even though they were always being kind (someone in my NCT group rumbled me and they were all nothing but supportive). I think a part of me felt that I was making the juggle of having a newborn and writing a regular column in a national newspaper look easy when, of course, it wasn't. In fact, I was only able to do it thanks to my husband, who took four months of parental leave, and because our baby ended up being partially formula fed. That, and the understanding and flexibility of my editors, who couldn't have been more supportive.

When I first went to my editor Kirsty Major with the idea for this series, she was not yet a mother herself, but she understood immediately what I meant when I said that I wanted to write about parenthood in a way that spoke to our generation, whether my readers decided to become parents or not. To my mind, my generation of twenty- and thirty-somethings were facing a particular range of challenges as we considered the possibilities of becoming parents – from housing, cost of living and climate crises, to shifting gender roles and employment structures. I wanted to speak to those experiences at a time when it felt that hardly anyone was doing so. And I wanted to be inclusive of family structures and sexualities of all kinds, including of those people who, for whatever reason, don't end up being parents. As friends who don't have kids have told me, not having your own doesn't mean that your life is absent of children, or that how they are raised is irrelevant to you. We all have a stake in the next generation, and our capacity for love goes beyond our immediate families.

Throughout this project, I have tried to be mindful of those who have different experiences to my own. No two families are the same, and the fact that we are seeing more tolerance and understanding of all these differences and life experiences can only be a good thing. A lot of mainstream parenting content not only assumed a nuclear, heterosexual family, but it also seemed to think everyone had the same level of middle-class wealth and comfort. I vividly remember looking at a feature in a newspaper about how to decorate a nursery, recommending a cot that cost more than £1,000. It made me feel awful. The rise of the influencer has only exacerbated this problem, and as a pregnant woman living in a rented flat, and as a daughter raised for the second half of her childhood by a skint single mother, none of it really spoke to me.

A lot of writing also assumed that everyone in the family was healthy. While writing, I kept in my heart, as much as possible, the thought of babies and children with health needs, neurodivergence and disabilities, and their families. Some of my friends had babies who were poorly or in hospital, and my brother is autistic, so I knew how it is to love a child who didn't smile, or speak at the same time as other babies, and what a worry it can be. I also knew there were other parents who had lost babies and, as a trauma response, had become hypervigilant about the health of their newborns.

This is why I didn't want to focus on developmental milestones – which have become more and more of a modern obsession – in a way that could make other parents feel worried, sad or excluded. There were times where the well-meaning but ableist attitudes of some other parents really got me down. The phrase 'They all walk and talk eventually' needs to be consigned to the dustbin.

Ultimately, parenting is a deeply personal experience and will be different for each and every one of us. There will be times when my words here do not speak directly to you, and you will vehemently disagree with me. There is no escaping that, but I hope that even if, say, you have a wonderful, easy time breastfeeding, my writing might help you understand that friend who is struggling with it. And I hope that those readers parenting solo, in same-sex relationships, or who do not have children will find themselves here, too.

I know that most people who read and buy this book will either be parents themselves or will be giving it as a gift to prospective or new parents. To you, I would like to offer a reminder that I am no expert: if parenthood has taught me anything, it is that none of us know what the hell we are doing. I hope that, whether you agree with me or find yourself throwing the book across the room, at least some of what it contains makes you feel less alone.

In writing these pieces, and the rest of this book, I have done my utmost to render the truth of my experience, without either scaremongering or putting on the rose-tinted glasses of hindsight. I'm not sure I've always succeeded in maintaining this balance but, nevertheless, I feel proud to have explored this tension. Other than the gift of becoming a mother to my son, writing about the experience has been one of my life's great joys.

For a few months after I had my son, I was unable to process the permanence of this change. Sometimes I would be overtaken by a sort of vertigo; it struck me one sunny day, as my son napped in his bassinet under a canopy of trees: 'My God, I am someone's mother – for ever.' If the transition to parenthood at times felt overwhelming, it was also laced with awe, and gratitude for being given the strongest attachment to another being that I have ever known. There was something so deeply primal about the ache in my breasts, or the feeling of waking up and groping the bedclothes around me for his tiny body. Once the madness of the hormones died down (they take two years to fully go back to normal), I felt a part of myself return to me. In many ways, I was the same person I had always been, but with one fundamental transformation: my centre of gravity had become, simply, him. I have come to think of this time as 'soul-shifting'.

Now, my tiny boy who couldn't wait, despite not being fully ready for the world, comes up past my waist. He no longer needs my body for sustenance, but he still needs it for comfort. As I knelt on the carpet this morning, he stood with his arms around me, his head buried in my shoulder. I marvelled at how time passes, and at the challenges we have overcome so far. There will be more to come, I know that, but we will be all right, because my soul has settled. When things are hard, just remember that yours will, too.

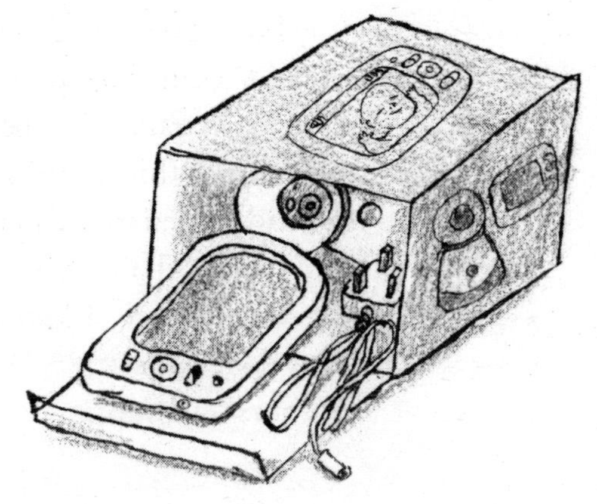

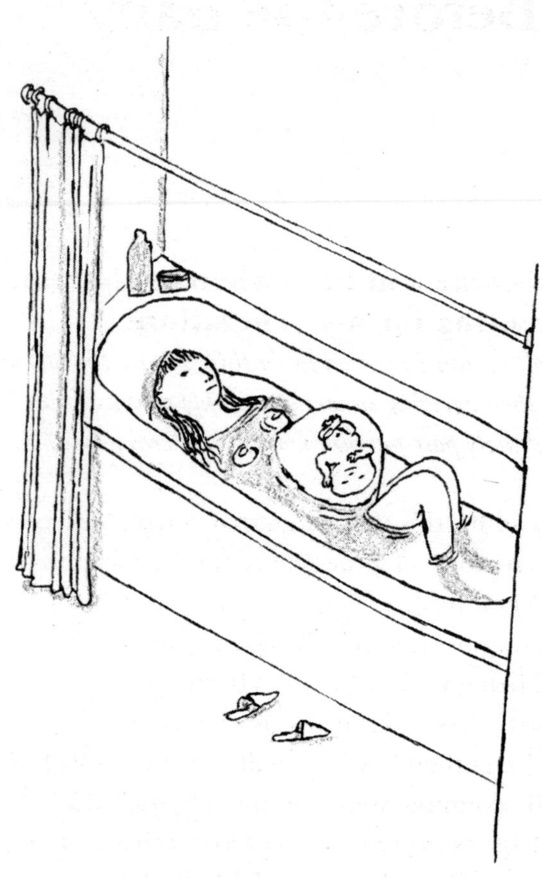

Before the Baby

I've just become a mum – where is the writing about parenting for my generation?

(Or: The whole reason I wanted to do this, despite the fact that pitching and then agreeing to write a weekly column from being almost immediately post-partum was quite a crazy idea)

If you are reading this, it means that I have just become a mother. For reasons of practicality, and superstition, I am writing this column in advance. I am currently twenty-nine weeks pregnant, just into my third trimester, but this will not run until, all being well, my baby is born.

Born, too – less painfully – is this column series, 'The Republic of Parenthood', which will hopefully speak to other parents, and examine some of the philosophical, political and cultural issues around modern parenthood. I chose the name to honour 'The Republic of Motherhood', a beautiful poem by Liz Berry that evokes the feeling of which many new mothers speak; of joining a new society, almost, which feels like a closed-off state separate from the rest of the world, one that necessitates the learning of new rules and customs:

I stood with my sisters in the queues of Motherhood –
the weighing clinic, the supermarket – waiting
for Motherhood's bureaucracies to open their doors.
As required, I stood beneath the flag of Motherhood
and opened my mouth although I did not know the anthem.

For Berry, the Republic of Motherhood is 'a wild queendom', and, though I feel her words deeply, I wanted this series to include fathers and families of all shapes and sizes. Hence: parenthood. I also chose the name semi-ironically, for though parenthood may feel like a separate state to some, we are all, ultimately, part of a collective, a community. It seems to be that problems arise when we fail to acknowledge the role parents play in that and – vice versa – the part played by those who are childless and childfree (two slightly different things, as I will come to explore). So I hope this series speaks too, to non-parents, and helps to foster solidarity between us all, whatever our choices.

It is easy to say that everything about pregnancy and motherhood has been written already, and certainly I am joining a crowded field. Accordingly, I promise not to write as though I am the first woman to ever have given birth to a child, nor can I really profess to know anything. I can be honest, but I cannot be didactic, because I am a complete novice.

This is all sounding rather earnest, so I also promise not to take myself too seriously. So much writing about parenthood feels to me to be po-faced, moralistic in tone, painfully middle-class and passé. Very little of it seems to speak to parents of my generation and younger, who face unique struggles in addition to all the usual challenges, during an unprecedented societal moment and with a moral panic about the birth rate humming in the background.

For example, last night I read a couple of newspaper articles that talked about home decoration for parents. Both assumed that everyone lives in a giant Victorian terrace, recommending lethally expensive furniture and accessories – cot canopies costing more than £100, a smart cot that 'sleep-trains' your baby, retailing at more than a grand – and featuring quotes from influencers and mummy bloggers. As someone who lives in a rented flat and, with the best will in the world, has zero interest in following these women, I thought there might be some writing out there that spoke to me during my pregnancy. But there was very little. And there must be others like me, who are spending their days in a state of near constant bemusement and frustration. Instead, I have turned to older female writers, to Rachel Cusk, Anne Enright, Maggie O'Farrell, Rebecca Walker, Adrienne Rich, Elena Ferrante and Audre Lorde, for inspiration.

It's been a strange time to be pregnant: in the middle of a pandemic, though at a stage, thankfully, when vaccines have been available. It has meant that, while others have returned to an approximation of normal life, those who are pregnant and their partners are still living in varying degrees of lockdown. Even when we've had the jab, the advice is to be extra careful, and no one wants to risk their baby's health or – should their partner catch Covid – risk them being unable to be present at the birth.

I have been lucky to have a pregnancy that has mostly been happy and healthy, but at times it has also felt curiously lonely. Reading and writing about it has helped, and I hope will continue to do so.

When I showed my mother the poem 'The Republic of Motherhood', she praised it, but she also said: 'It isn't like this, you know, for everyone.' It was my first glimpse of a gulf between those who have struggled in parenthood, and those who have thrived. I have friends in both camps, and at this stage have no idea where I will fall: perhaps, like many people, somewhere in between.

This is why it is important to stress that I do not believe my experience to be that of anyone else, and the purpose of this column is not to alienate, but to include. Our experiences may all be different, but we have much in common, whether we are parents or are contemplating parenthood, or have decided against it, or crave it desperately only to be thwarted. Wherever you fall, I hope this column speaks to you. And I hereby promise that I will never subject you to a single anecdote about changing my baby's nappy. Well, not unless it's really, really funny.

To have a child or not is a huge decision. So why is there so little discussion of it?

(Or, can people please stop saying you have to be 100 per cent sure before you have a baby?)

Long before I became pregnant, I would ask people how they knew that they wanted to have children. Was there a lightning moment, or had the longing grown and grown until it became too much to ignore? Of course, the answers I got were as varied as people themselves. Some were able to distil it into a clear instant: taking hold of a small child's hand for the first time, or seeing a baby on a bus one day and knowing, suddenly. Others were influenced by life events: the death of a parent was a common one, leading them to reflect on how bloodlines unfurl, wanting to see a little of that beloved parent manifest in a new being. Others had always known, in their bones, since their own childhoods.

Then, for women, there was the so-called biological clock. Not so much a desire for a child, but an awareness that time could be running out, and a sort of not-wanting, a double negative: not-wanting to have not had a child. Many of these women expressed guilt at not having felt 'the longing', as though an innate-seeming, visceral dose of baby fever was the norm, and, in their absence of strong maternal feelings, they were deviating from it. But it does not seem that way to me, and besides, my own feelings were far from simple. At times it felt as though my body was at war with my brain. There were so many rational reasons not to become a parent, and yet the longing I felt was so powerful that it was making me unspeakably sad not to be.

I say 'body', but of course I don't know. I can write only of how it felt, but scientifically, the jury remains out on whether the desire for parenthood is down to nature or nurture, and both biology and culture are likely to contribute. We are social animals, and social pressure can be enormous. I like to think that I was immune to this, though during 2020–21 it felt as though everyone I knew was having a baby, except me. I sat on the sidelines, wanting it, but dithering.

It is, of course, a privilege to dither. Before the advent of contraception, becoming a parent couldn't really be described as a decision at all. Perhaps this is why my search for historical sources that showed women interrogating the question was rather fruitless. Even speaking to women of older generations, who came of age post-contraception, there's a sense that there wasn't much thought given to the question. 'It's just what you did', is a sentence that came up time and time again, and several older women have expressed their admiration for my generation for taking the prospect so seriously.

Role models are also a factor. My mother has quite a few friends who are childfree, and so I never grew up believing that motherhood was destiny. I knew that there were many kinds of life that one could have, and also that I could have a relationship with children in other ways: as an aunt, a godparent, a friend. In fact, I found that the decision to be childfree was far better documented than the decision to become a parent. It feels as though there is still a taboo when it comes to expressing having had entirely rational doubts about becoming a parent, only to go ahead and take the plunge. I have lost count of the number of times that I have read that you should only do so if you are '100 per cent sure'. As someone who, for a variety of reasons, has never been 100 per cent sure about anything in my life, that feels pretty shaming.

It feels to me as though we need more open conversations about the decision-making process, and better ways of supporting people who are in the midst of it. We are surrounded by panic about the birth rate – for the first time in history, half the women in England and Wales have not had a child by the time they reach thirty, yet there still seems to be little exploration of the fact that many Western countries are what could be termed hostile environments for new parents. There are many reasons – economic, educational, environmental – why a person may delay parenthood, and my generation and those younger face unprecedented hardships. On top of that, there is evidence to suggest that women are happier without children and a spouse. When a happiness expert spoke about this in 2019, people were enraged, but the fact remains that the sexist balance of domestic labour makes a lot of women miserable, and who can blame them for choosing another path?

As with anything to do with parenthood, we could do with less judgement, and more listening. And perhaps, as Sheila Heti suggests in her novel *Motherhood*, the constant questioning is all 'a huge conspiracy to keep women in their thirties – when you finally have some brains and some skills and experience – from doing anything useful with them at all'.

'Enjoy it while you can'. Is there a more gloomy phrase to hear while pregnant?

(Or: For the love of God, stop scaring the hell out of expectant parents)

'Enjoy it while you can': how I've come to dislike these five little words, which have followed me everywhere since my pregnancy became obvious. Suddenly, they are applied to anything pleasurable – sleep, holidays, a meal in a restaurant. 'Enjoy it while you can,' people say (because when the baby comes, your life as you know it will be over).

They mean well, I think, but I'll confess that I've been shocked by the negativity surrounding parenthood. People seem to feel that they simply must tell you how hard it is, warts and all, maybe because no one told them, and they do it with the zeal of missionaries: they have seen the truth, and it is terrible to behold. Hollie McNish has a book of poetry about parenthood called *Nobody Told Me*. Mine would be called *Everybody Told Me, All the Time, Until I Had to Ask Them to Stop.*

Before I had the baby, it's not that I thought parenthood was going to be a breeze – I just wanted to hear a tiny bit of positive feedback about it.

During pregnancy you realise pretty quickly that, for your own sanity, you will need to avoid certain subjects. In the early months, tales of miscarriage seemed to be everywhere (and this is after all the tales of fertility woe, which, in my case anyway, led to the belief that it would be near-impossible to get pregnant). If you get to twelve weeks, suddenly stories about foetal anomalies seem to spring up. And after that it's stillbirths, traumatic labours, sepsis, death. I found myself desperate to read a story along the lines of: 'Woman conceives child naturally, only to carry and give birth to said child without complications.'

This is not to be flippant about the very real suffering of many women, which for decades was cloaked in shameful silence. Pregnancy and birth can be dangerous and traumatising, particularly for women but also for men. Part of the reason that we are seeing these stories now is because the cult of motherhood positivity felt so suffocating. Among my friendship group are women and their partners who have suffered traumatic births, pregnancy loss and postnatal depression. Some people have become parents during the pandemic, with all of the unique challenges that poses. I have listened to their testimonies and, I hope, supported them. These conversations are often long and nuanced, and feature moments of joy as well as pain. They perhaps reflect better the experience of parenthood than many articles are able to.

No, it is the strangers who seem to present the most negativity. It is as though they think pregnant women are wandering blindly into parenthood and must be shown the light. The implication is that before embarking on this journey, we lived carefree existences without responsibility. But this is not the reality for everyone: for example, when I was a child I was a carer for my brother. Others will have nursed loved ones through illness and death, or supported them through periods of mental illness. It may not be an identical experience to that of being a parent, but there are many ways to care, and to express that care. Others who are childfree exercise their caring impulses through their family and community networks, through fostering, volunteering, political activism. Or perhaps, snotty as the Pope has been about this, they care for animals. We are all a part of a collective of which caring is a crucial aspect.

At least, that's how I see it. Some frame parenthood as a dividing line – on the one side those who embark upon it, on the other those who don't. But I've never seen it that way: I prefer to choose solidarity.

People often say that when you are pregnant, you become public property. In *Making Babies*, Anne Enright writes of how, during her pregnancy, she felt she became a sort of vessel for other people's projections. 'Everyone's unconscious was very close to their mouth,' she writes. 'Whatever my pregnant body triggered was not political, or social, it was animal and ancient and quite helpless.'

Perhaps, in all the parenting negativity, we are seeing an overcorrection. An attempt to be more honest about the challenges that has spilled over into a tide that, at times, can feel overwhelming, especially to those who are prone to anxiety or have suffered from mental illness. I found myself clinging to the stories of those few strangers who smiled at my news and told me of their parenting joys: the cabby who picked me up from my first midwife appointment and told me how much he loves being a dad; the woman on holiday who vividly described nursing her son, how his little dark eyes would lock with hers so that they felt like the only two people in the world. Whenever I heard another 'Enjoy it while you can', I held on to these snippets and tried not to panic.

What worked

- Even though I decided motherhood was for me, I found the 2015 essay collection *Selfish, Shallow, and Self-Absorbed: Sixteen Writers on the Decision Not to Have Kids* fascinating, especially as it included men, one of whom (Geoff Dyer), as the *New York Times* reviewer pointed out, shows 'what it looks like to have a relationship to the topic that is completely unburdened by guilt or self-doubt.'

- Ginger and incredibly spicy food. My morning sickness remedies.

- I found that pregnancy pillows are worth the money. I found lying down so uncomfortable that I hardly slept for the last couple of months of my pregnancy. I tried shoring myself up with piles of feather pillows, but the only thing that seemed to truly give my aching hips and back some relief was a pregnancy pillow (mine was from BellaMoon, and is like a giant, squishy croissant that you straddle, supporting you to sleep on your side). It isn't cheap and takes up roughly the same space in the bed as a person, but it worked.

- Crodino, an Italian non-alcoholic aperitif. This is essential for any pregnant woman who normally likes a negroni or spritz. I found Nozeco and other non-alcoholic wine brands horrifically sweet, so this was my beverage of choice. Lucky Saint was my preferred non-alcoholic beer, but the Corona and Birra Moretti ones are also not bad, either.

- Hypnobirthing. I initially put this in the 'what's not working' section of my column, because many of the 'positive birth stories' were along the following lines: 'During my home birth, I was bleeding out all over the living room floor. The midwife recommended that I go to hospital, but, using what I learned in hypnobirthing, I resisted all attempts at medical intervention.' I still have mixed feelings about hypnobirthing, especially the way in which some less scrupulous practitioners put the blame for a difficult birth on a woman's fear and anxiety, when we know that every birth is unique and that many complications are unavoidable. I wish there wasn't such a stigma against pain relief and intervention in these circles, as the culture of 'normal birth at all costs' can have tragic consequences, as reports such as the 2022 Ockenden Maternity Review have shown. But hypnobirthing did help keep me calm during a difficult point in my labour when pain relief was not forthcoming, and for that I am grateful.

- Epidurals. There should be a statue to the person who invented them – Fidel Pagés, a Spanish surgeon, in 1921, in case you're interested – outside every labour ward in the country.

- The Adagietto from Mahler's Fifth Symphony. My mum recommended that I play a piece of music to my baby in the womb as a way of soothing him. I chose this on her recommendation, not only because it's beautiful, but because it lasts for the perfect amount of time to lull a baby to sleep. As my mum predicted, once he was out of the womb I only had to play this to him, and he would drop off. Even now, as he approaches the age of three, it has the ability to calm him. Miraculous.

What didn't

- Maternity clothing. I was lucky in that I didn't have to buy a whole new wardrobe, so made the most of my stretchiest clothes, plus H&M maternity leggings (excellent). I did occasionally go in search of maternity wear, though, and always came away feeling disillusioned. Even brands like Seraphine felt a bit square, as though being pregnant meant suddenly having to dress as conventionally as possible. In the end I resorted to second-hand Topshop maternity (RIP) pieces from Vinted, but there remains a gap in the market.

- Baths. I had the most appalling bath while heavily pregnant. It was lukewarm, as medically recommended (I used my husband's homebrew thermometer to check it was below 37°C). I thought I'd try the whole of Mahler's Fifth Symphony, not realising how bellicose and bombastic it was. 'Are you OK in there?' my husband asked, as I sat in a cold bath listening to a cacophony of trumpets. 'You sound like you should be piloting a Spitfire.'

- I found myself hating the tone of a lot of pregnancy books targeted at women, which was infantilising and identity-sapping. I disliked being referred to as a disembodied 'mum', and language such as 'lady garden' and 'sore parts' made me want to scream. As for some of the advice, a section on the idea of 'freedom Friday' – which sees a husband deign to give his wife one 'night off' a week, followed by 'top tips on how not to hate your partner' made me wonder if I had entered a wormhole straight to the 1950s. Sadly, barbiturates were not suggested as a remedy.

- Packed off to triage with high blood pressure that turned out to be caused by white coat syndrome, I saw a woman's waters break in the waiting room. 'Oh shit,' she said, 'my trackies.' She was put in the bay next to mine. 'This is the most pain I have ever been in,' she yelled, ensuring my blood pressure remained as high as ever. 'They do say that labour is painful,' her partner said, as we each contemplate ways in which we would kill him. 'I mean, that shouldn't come as a surprise. They do tell you that, babe.' Birth partners: just because you're thinking it, doesn't mean you should say it.

- The medical examination lights at the hospital. Instead, they were examining patients in labour with these giant black battery-operated torches, of the sort that you might take caving. A depressing indictment of the underfunding of the NHS, but it did give me a good laugh at a scary time.

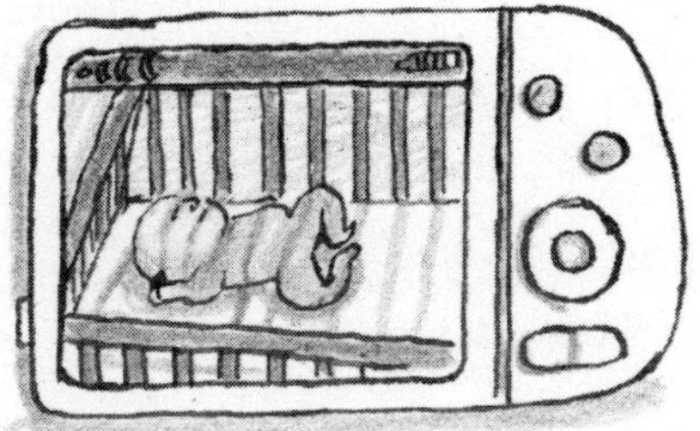

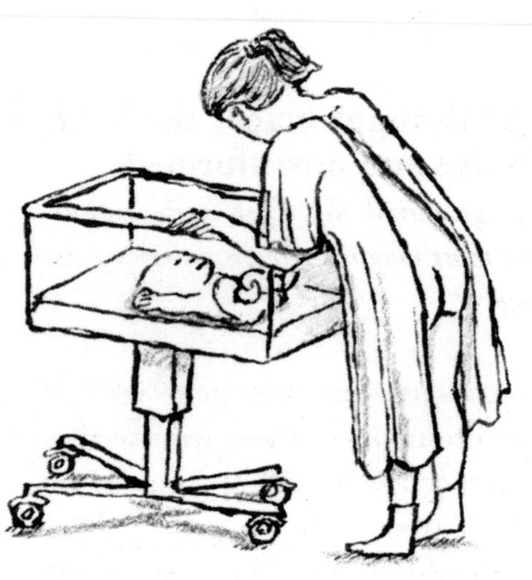

0–3 months

Everything I thought before the birth of my son now feels naive and misinformed

(Or: In which I give birth five weeks early, and am reeling from the shock of the most magnificent, insane thing that has ever happened to me)

I had been supposed to file two more columns in this series in advance, before taking some leave, but five weeks ago my waters broke in spectacular fashion – the way they do in films, the way the NCT woman said you really didn't want them to break. 'It's too early,' I kept saying, again like some cinema cliché. During the rush to the hospital, our Uber got stuck behind a hearse travelling at a suitably funereal pace. The catastrophist in me assumed an omen. The writer in me rolled her eyes and thought: nice touch.

And so the boy is here (bairn is not a word I ever used before, but for some reason I cannot stop, as though my northern ancestors have risen up in me, conjured by all the drama). I am still adjusting to the fact that he is no longer inside me, that I thought I had five more weeks of kicks and punches, how I never got to see the reverse imprint of his hand on my skin. Anxieties about Covid notwithstanding, I loved being pregnant with him, and we've been catapulted into the fourth trimester without quite being done with the third. He is here and hardly anything is ready, and, despite needing some help from some magnificent doctors, he is all right, and my life is transformed.

My colleague Eva Wiseman was right about the love feeling two centimetres from grief. I have been skinned alive. I weep at the merest trifle, as if I'm the baby. On the night we came home from hospital, I cried and cried. I want a bumper between my new family and the world. I could have done without Billy Bragg's 'Tank Park Salute' coming on the radio in the kitchen: another microwave meal salted with tears. The love feels like terror too: of all the ways in which he could be taken from me (it's the women who are blasé that we worry about, said the discharging midwife).

But most of all, it feels like gratitude. For him: my dream come true. For his father. For the medical care, the costs of which in another place would have run, possibly, into the millions. For our safety. The day after I had him, the Russians bombed a Ukrainian maternity hospital. Before my son's arrival, I had been reading of the women giving birth underground. 'Don't look at the news,' a friend texted, as I lay in a bay without my baby, who had been rushed to neonatal intensive care, listening to the sounds of labouring women, and she was right. I could not bear it.

How to articulate the transfiguration from not-mother to mother? I am the same person, and yet everything I wrote before feels naive and misinformed. It is as though I have been made party to some great secret. As though, when I stepped out of that taxi and into the old, looming Victorian building, with its ghost sign saying 'Women's Receiving

Ward', just as my own mother and thousands of other women had before me, I was initiated. Though that could, of course, be the drugs.

I didn't have a birth plan. I was due to have a scan, to meet the obstetrician to discuss the best way forward. The hypnobirthing book I bought second-hand in an attempt to calm my fears regarding childbirth was clear in its views of the sort of delivery I should have. I am not so impressionable, and, when I skipped forward to read about the aftermath, the page proclaiming: 'You've birthed a baby and you're a goddamn goddess', in a register I have come to dislike, was decorated with – I kid you not – a smear of what looked like blood. Disgusting, but you could say it was the most honest thing in the entire book. There was, indeed, blood.

During my week in the hospital, I kept seeing glimpses through windows of the most beautiful spring skies, promising a world outside for the both of us, if he would only breathe and feed on his own. After a few days I realised that I was not a prisoner; I could go out for a walk. In the lift I joked with a man about a discarded hat and how gross it would be if one of us put it on, and I was grateful that I could still hold a conversation that was not about my baby.

At the same time, he is everything, just as I am to him. My boy who could not wait, but whose eyes are scarcely open. Love, in the words of Sylvia Plath, set him going like a 'fat gold watch', but it has taken far more treatment than a 'slap on the soles' from a midwife to give him a healthy start in life.

In the small hours, in the bluish darkness of the ward, I sat next to his incubator and tried to remember lullabies, but amid the fear and the love and the painkiller fog the words had all vanished. Instead, as the machines beeped reassuringly and I stroked his skin through the small porthole, no longer able to be the ship that carried him, he got 'Here Comes the Sun'.

Turns out breastfeeding really does hurt – why does no one tell you?

(Or: How the hardest part of the fourth trimester was, for me, the thing I least expected)

I never thought breastfeeding would be hard. When I thought about it at all, my mind conjured beatific scenes suffused with a sort of religious glow. There I was, genteelly offering the child a nipple in the manner of a renaissance Madonna, which the child accepted politely and cherubically. What a pretty picture we made.

Well, those preconceptions were – excuse my language – complete horseshit. These days I envisage more of a triptych: the infant Jesus spluttering at the breast, face purple with hangry fury; the infant Jesus posseting milk down Mary's front; the infant Jesus and the nappy explosion.

A few weeks ago, I wrote about the negativity surrounding parenthood, and how people love to bombard pregnant women with it. The only exception I'd make to this is breastfeeding. Breastfeeding has incredible PR. You're told constantly how amazing it is for you and the baby. It's the best way to nourish and bond with your child, who will become a genius as a result! It's so convenient! You'll lose so much weight! Most importantly, it's hugely beneficial to the baby's health!

No one says: it hurts. At least not beforehand. Once you tell other mothers it hurts they say, grimly, 'yep'. It makes sense that it would hurt, because having a small creature attacking your nipples every forty minutes would hurt, wouldn't it? It's OK though, because, you're told, they'll 'toughen up'. Tough nipples: just what I always wanted.

Meanwhile, if you tell professionals that it hurts they will tell you that you're doing it wrong, which makes it feel worse. (Maybe you are doing it wrong – historically, you'd be surrounded by experienced female relatives who would help position you and the baby correctly.) Perhaps you already feel like enough of a failure, because desperately wanting to feed your child with your body and not being able to taps into something quite fundamental, really. Something that may have the potential to make you depressed.

The UK has one of the lowest breastfeeding rates in the world, with just 24 per cent of women exclusively breastfeeding at six weeks in England and 1 per cent at six months, which is recommended by the WHO. Eight out of ten women stopped before they wanted to. Furthermore, while breastfeeding is linked to lower rates of postnatal depression, a large-scale survey also found that women who wanted to breastfeed but did not (or could not) were over twice as likely to become depressed as mothers who had not planned to, and who did not, breastfeed.

I'm not surprised. The culture of guilt – much of which manifests in subtle, almost diffuse atmospheric pressure, though social media obnoxiousness also plays a role – makes me want to smash things, but I'm too tired. Breastfeeding, I read, is the equivalent of walking seven miles a day. Another thing they don't tell you is that you might not ever get more than three hours' sleep, none of it deep. And you'll realise how profoundly uncomfortable your sofa is.

I can see why they don't want to put women off, what with the enormous public health benefits of breastfeeding, for babies especially. Besides, many women have a fine old time of it. They are 'EBF' – exclusively breastfeeding – a phrase I've started to imagine accompanied by jazz hands. Some post photographs of all the milk they are expressing and freezing – look! So much milk! Their proud tallies: fourteen months! eighteen months!

thirty-six months! And they should be proud. It's work. I find myself thinking about the wet nurses throughout history who would take in extra infants to feed as well as their own. The labour involved would have been intensely physically and emotionally draining. I also sympathise a bit more with the women who chose to outsource it than I perhaps once did.

Saying all this, when it starts to go well, it's lovely, and if your baby isn't premature and you don't have to deal with tongue tie, undersupply, oversupply, mastitis or blocked ducts it might be a very simple, very peaceful, happy process. I've been mostly very lucky with the support I've received with the challenges of feeding a pre-term baby, but others have not been so fortunate. There is something wrong with a culture wherein the mother's sanity can be sidelined to the extent that – as one parent and psychologist described – the only professional who might tell a woman that it's OK to give her baby formula is part of a perinatal mental health team. Promotion of breastfeeding, important though it is, should never come at the expense of a mother's mental health. To quote one expert: 'Breastmilk does not care for, nurture and bond with the baby. A mother does.'

Meanwhile, my friend who has had a double mastectomy is irritated that there's a law prohibiting the discounting of infant formula. She also, having observed the culture of guilt, says she feels glad the decision how to feed her baby was taken out of her hands. Think on that statement for a moment.

As it is, my own 'breastfeeding journey' (another phrase I hate) has involved a rail replacement bus. I'm grateful for the existence of formula for keeping my baby alive when I couldn't, and for helping my baby grow to a healthy size while I established breastfeeding. I'm not about to become a shill for big formula, who have behaved despicably in all kinds of ways, but nor will I self-flagellate. Or I'll try not to, at least not all the time.

As for advice from all the self-appointed freelance paediatricians, I can do without it. A good lactation consultant, though, is worth her weight in gold. Turns out, with the right support, it can get better – as it has for us. It's a shame that so many British women lack that support after years of government cuts.

There are a multitude of reasons why a woman might stop breastfeeding, including a lack of support, needing to work, pathetic paternity leave provision (having a partner who can feed the mother while she feeds the baby is a luxury few have), the stigmatising of public feeding, or mental health concerns. Guilt-tripping parents who are struggling or hiding the challenges of breastfeeding from them will not solve, and may even worsen, the problem.

Having a baby has been a tornado through my life – I see why new parents dream of communes

(Or: It hits me how modern society isn't equipped to support new parents)

The nuclear family is ill suited to effective childrearing. This should be news to no one. Yet when my mum said it, having taken the baby from me so that I could – finally – shower off myriad effluences, I felt it in my bones. Even though my husband has been at home on shared parental leave and has been doing all the cooking and laundry, and half the feeding (a luxury few can afford), I calculate that each newborn needs at least three, possibly four, adults to bring things up to a level beyond 'just about coping'.

And yet the situation if you're in a heterosexual pairing is that, after two weeks, most men go back to work and their partners are home alone with a baby in an endless cycle of feeding, sleeping and defecating, trying to time it so that they can actually exit the house and see another human being before the next circle of hell begins.

'What's it like?' a friend asked me, of motherhood. 'It's like a tornado crashing through the middle of your life,' I said, 'so you wake up in Oz and everything's in Technicolor. But also, you've been crushed by a house.'

Thank heavens, then, for grandparents, and if you're lucky enough to live close to them (and they are willing to help) you have won the childcare lottery. The love one has for one's grandchildren is in some ways purer, less complicated, a grandmother recently told me, and certainly less guilt-ridden. At the root of it is the Darwinian knowledge that you would step in if anything happened to the parents, she said. Not so long ago, women regularly did not make it through childbirth alive, after all.

Likewise, anyone who brings you food in the early weeks takes on god-level status. Where hunter-gatherers used to be, instead there's a website called Take Them a Meal, which allows friends to coordinate the logistics. Fidelity to humanity's tribal, mutually supportive origins may have been all but obliterated by the Industrial Revolution and the rise of capitalism, but we do have online deliveries. Hence cheese platters sent by friends in Brooklyn and Somerset, and fruit and champagne courtesy of my sister-in-law in New Zealand. My aunt Teresa, meanwhile, has been trekking over once a week with a full meal that she has prepared. The first week that we came home from hospital with our pre-term baby, she brought us a full roast chicken dinner with lemon pudding for after, complete with a little jam jars of gravy and cream respectively. I could have cried (I did cry).

So I understand why new parents – mothers especially – have confided in me that they have found themselves fantasising about communes (and not in a sexual way, that's what got us all in this mess in the first place). Our fragmented society makes childcare a lonely and expensive business, especially when you've gravitated to a city. I was born into a shared co-operative house containing eight adults, two of whom were East German defectors sleeping on the living room floor. My mother said it was great to have other adults to talk to. For many, days on maternity leave seem to stretch out endlessly, and friends say it can feel like you've achieved little while your partner has been at work. (The book *What Mothers Do: Especially When It Looks Like Nothing* is brilliant at taking such beliefs to task.) So many women spending so much time alone with their babies without family support could exacerbate postnatal depression.

Though we live far from our extended families, I have been bowled over by the love and kindness we've received, such as my mother-in-law picking up last-minute sleepsuits that didn't swamp our premature baby. My thoughts have turned to immigrant women, some of whom have emailed me about their experiences, trying to make it through without their family networks. In some cultures it is the norm, postpartum, for the woman to take to her bed to feed the baby while a deluge of relatives descend to care for her. I've also been thinking of the new parents who were robbed of contact with their families during the pandemic, but who say they at least found solace in the cocoon they were able to form at home thanks to fathers working from home.

The proverb 'it takes a village to raise a child' is often cited to new parents, but in much of the West we seem to have turned our backs on childrearing as a collective endeavour. It is instead the business of individuals, who must shoulder the burden in their atomised units, subject to the twin forces of extortionate childcare and pathetic paid paternity-leave provision.

Yet the traditional heterosexual nuclear family is on its way out: among my friends are gay couples who have conceived thanks to surrogacy or IVF, blended families, co-parents, single parents and women in traditional marriages, who are basically single parents and will continue to be so, once they inevitably divorce their husbands. Perhaps it's time to dismantle it even further or, rather, expand our understanding of it. I have never wanted my village more, and never have they felt so far away.

A third of new mothers are traumatised by childbirth, but there's one easy way to help

(Or: How my dear friend found the words to talk about birth trauma)

Jessica Cornwell was silent in labour. During the forceps and ventouse delivery of her twins she haemorrhaged, and her life was saved by a doctor who inserted their hand into her womb to remove her placenta. One of her sons was rushed to the newborn intensive care unit. 'I couldn't talk,' she writes in *Birth Notes*, her memoir of recovery from the post-traumatic stress disorder (PTSD) she developed. 'I couldn't say anything at all.'

Cornwell now knows that she entered a dissociative state during the birth. 'I started dissociating pretty much the minute that I went into labour, and a lot of the midwives commented on how quiet I was. How I handled pain well,' she tells me. Her book, a visceral, poetic account of her journey to diagnosis and treatment, and a damning indictment of the lack of knowledge of, and research into, birth trauma, was originally going to be called *Where There Are No Words*.

I've been thinking a lot about words and language since I gave birth, how good communication can save a person from becoming traumatised. Mental health professionals tell me that it is often when patients (and their birth partners) feel that communication has been poor, when they have no idea what is happening to them or to their body, that PTSD symptoms can result. 'Intense fear tends to be one of the main causes of PTSD, and so, if she feels that everything is out of control, no one is telling her what's happening, no one is listening to her, all of that combined can cause PTSD,' says Dr Kim Thomas of the Birth Trauma Association. 'A lot of women will say "I thought my baby was about to die" or they think that they are about to die, but none of the hospital staff seem to be cognisant of this.'

According to one study, every third woman would describe their experience of giving birth as traumatic, yet until relatively recently childbirth wasn't considered an event that could cause PTSD. It was normal, natural. According to the *Diagnostic and Statistical Manual of Mental Disorders 3*, PTSD was the result of events that were 'generally outside the range of usual human experience'. This was only removed in 2013, and childbirth is still not explicitly listed as a potential stressor, though experts are finally in agreement that it can be.

Nevertheless, birth trauma is often misdiagnosed as postnatal depression. It took Cornwell two years to get her diagnosis, having been told she had postnatal depression, and again, where there should have been language there was instead an absence. Birth trauma and pregnancy simply weren't included on the 'life events' checklist she was given. She found herself wondering if 'the absence of traumatic categories related to motherhood was accidental, an oversight, or a deliberate omission – or if the research simply hasn't caught up yet'.

Watching Cornwell, who is a close friend, undergo her quest to put these experiences into words has been awe-inspiring. She is not alone in this. Sometimes it is several wines down, told almost in the style of a stand-up routine. At other times it is mentioned almost casually, like the occasion when a woman in a cafe handed me a coffee and gestured at the child in the playground opposite. 'I only have one,' she said, 'because they took my womb out afterwards.'

Finding the words, building a narrative, is what helps processing. I have received an outpouring of emails from women with birth trauma, often long, detailed accounts using medical terminology. These are women who have asked to see their notes so that they can work out what has happened to them, or who have attended debriefings. Always, the questions are the same: 'Why wasn't I listened to?'; 'Why did no one tell me what was happening?'; 'Why were my requests for pain relief ignored?' (asking for pain relief and not being granted it is a recurring theme); 'Why was this done to me without consent?'

Sometimes there are serious failings of care, but often it seems a traumatic birth is characterised by such communication gaps. Cornwell stresses that raising awareness of birth trauma is not about demonising overworked medical professionals, but working out how to improve the experience of birth for future patients so that we don't have to hear these stories time and time again. Entering a dissociative state, as she did, is a signpost of future PTSD, as is previous trauma such as sexual violence. She thinks that training to help doctors and midwives identify women who are unusually silent in labour so that they can be given help grounding them if they are dissociating could be a positive development. Thomas highlights a study in which women who were extra vulnerable had a 'psychology alert' sticker placed on their birth notes to make medical staff aware of mental health concerns, with great success. Staff can be coached in listening skills, and more professionals have been coming to them asking for training.

I'm still making my way through the birth stories that I have been sent. Each is unique, but there are some statements that could apply to all the women writing, such as this from a mother of three who almost died during her labour and is now living with lifelong health issues: 'The main thing that upsets me the most is that I had no voice. I wasn't listened to and I wasn't heard.'

Writing honestly about motherhood still provokes anger, but we must tell our stories

(Or: Why this column exists, for those that have derided it)

I've been thinking a lot about Rachel Cusk, specifically her memoir, *A Life's Work*, which turned twenty last year. The public reaction to this brilliant account of early motherhood was at the time swift and brutal – and the judgement it received came mostly from other women, writing in newspapers. Reading about it made me nervous to be straying into similar territory.

Having co-written a book in my twenties criticising women's magazines, I have been bitten by the fangs of public 'feminist' discourse before, most notably perhaps by Germaine Greer, whose assertion in her review that 'the female breast does not express unless compressed', has also been on my mind, as I leak through yet another three layers of fabric and laugh.

But nevertheless, I persisted, convinced that the fields Cusk embarked on were by this stage well ploughed. To read *A Life's Work* nowadays is to wonder what exactly was so controversial about it. Cusk's baby cries all the time, and she is upfront about how challenging this is and the loss of identity that motherhood entails. Much of what she writes is very funny: 'My grasp of the baby's calorific intake, hours of sleep, motor development and patterns of crying is professorial, while the rest of my life resembles a deserted settlement, an abandoned building in which a rotten timber occasionally breaks and comes crashing to the floor, scattering mice.'

Perhaps largely because of Cusk, honesty about motherhood is not as taboo as it once was (though lines such as 'pregnancy begins to seem to me more and more of a lie, a place populated by evangelicals and moralists and control freaks' still provoke a gasp of pleasure in their excoriating resonance). I have been pleasantly surprised by the reaction to my column so far. The letters and messages I have received have been deeply moving and have made me feel part of a community in these early days of my parenting journey.

Still, I keep wondering: what was it about *A Life's Work* that made the backlash so furious? For one thing, projection. As Cusk has noted, people judged the book not as readers, but as mothers. In a 2008 essay, she wrote: 'I was accused of child-hating, of postnatal depression, of shameless greed, of irresponsibility, of pretentiousness, of selfishness, of doom-mongering and, most often, of being too intellectual.' Its erudition is clearly part of it. It does not do to be too intelligent about motherhood. It undermines a deeply held notion that it is the preserve of instinct, that mothers dwell in a place of ingrained nurturing, and that to critique it is unnatural.

Provocative, too, is Cusk's refusal to caveat her sentences with statements such as 'but of course I love my child'. I, similarly, have resisted this, and so have had a mild taste of a similar medicine from readers who have said that I should be 'enjoying my baby'. It is true that I have not felt the need to wax lyrical about him – there is enough sentimental writing around motherhood as it is. Perhaps I need to state in print that, obviously, I love my baby to a degree that feels like a sort of madness, that I can bring myself to tears at the thought of anything happening to him. Yet it is not good writing; like much relating to motherhood, it has all been said before.

Older women are, in the main part, forgiving of a new mother's tendency to exclaim 'nobody told me!' but not all, as I discovered recently. The accusation that we do not listen to older women's experience because of ageism is, I think, misplaced. As Cusk, who was shocked and unprepared for motherhood, writes, there is a 'tone-deafness … with which a non-parent is afflicted when a parent speaks ... which leads us to wonder in bemusement why we were never told ... what parenthood was like'. Her own mother didn't tell her, because she couldn't remember (there is something to this – even friends whose babies are still young have struggled to recall much about the early weeks). Cusk says she dealt with the prospect of childbirth through 'denial', while noting that other women were rather quiet: 'except one, who told me that at one point she begged the midwife to shoot her'.

Thankfully, there seems less of a (to my mind, and Cusk's, dishonest) taboo against complaint than there was. These days, there are almost too many warts-and-all accounts, to the point that you find yourself craving positivity. And yet I am grateful for them, because I could not say I was not prepared. I embarked on motherhood fully cognisant of the sacrifices it would involve. I had been part of a community of mothers long before I became one, and I had done my reading.

And yet motherhood is not an exam that one sits. We should reserve the right to spend our pre-motherhood days thinking of it scarcely at all, a freedom the women of the past were never granted. Nor should we feel the need to constantly bow and scrape to those who have been there before: even discounting Covid, having a baby in 2022 is necessarily different to doing so in 2002, or 1992. We have the right to tell our own stories.

Besides, there's a reason people say that nothing prepares you. To know something intellectually is not the same as knowing it bodily. While pregnant, I read Anne Enright saying, of breastfeeding – the pain of which is one of the few things that has surprised me so far – that it 'fucking hurts'. Did I forget? Perhaps. But I think it is more likely that to feel such pain is so fundamentally different to reading about it.

In the best passage in *A Life's Work*, Cusk describes the experience of reading books that she has loved again since becoming a mother, and finding them changed. Suddenly they contain 'prophecies of what was to come, pictures of the very place in which I now stand'. 'I wonder how I could have read so much and learned so little,' she writes, having previously refuted the notion that you have to experience to understand.

Perhaps that is the lesson we should take to writing about motherhood: that it will always be shocking, and that its central conflicts, though in some ways perennial, are also products of our unique places in history. Which is why those who have trod the path before should be generous to new mothers. I certainly plan to be. And I suspect that Cusk, who has suffered more judgement than perhaps any other writer of motherhood, will be too.

What worked

- The Elvie breast pump, which enabled me to feed my pre-term baby. It sits silently inside your bra, and unlike other pumps it allows you to move around while wearing it, so you feel less like a cow being milked. It's expensive but it still feels as though it was worth it, especially in a situation such as ours, where we were initially separated and establishing breastfeeding was more difficult. A truly liberating invention.

- The book *DON'T PANIC! All the Stuff the Expectant Dad Needs to Know* by George Lewis. Unlike most parenting books, it features contributions from comedians including Elis James, Romesh Ranganathan and Josh Widdicombe, and it is very funny – not that my husband got to finish it in time.

- Caroline Walker's beautiful paintings of birth and early motherhood made me feel seen during pregnancy and those first wild nights.

- Ewan the Dream Sheep, a cuddly cartoon sheep that glows red and plays womb-like sounds (yes, really) to help babies drift off to sleep. Millions have been sold and I can understand why, because it seems to have miraculous soporific effects.

- Multi-Mam nipple compresses. When breastfeeding is sore, these are a miracle remedy. They cost more than other brands, but they are far more soothing and cooling. The Weleda balm is also fantastic.

- Breastfeeding tea really did seem to increase my supply. My cousin – a breastfeeding counsellor – also recommended chocolate and oats for helping to increase supply, so I basically lived off M&S Belgian milk chocolate dipped flapjacks, which I still haven't forgiven them for discontinuing.

What didn't

- Cotton buds. We were told to eschew wipes and lotions and that all we needed to wipe the baby's bum were cotton buds and water, plus a bit of olive oil if they had nappy rash. We didn't even make it out of the hospital before we jettisoned this. All the cotton buds seemed to do was spread the poo around, while the doctors and nurses in the NICU were smearing fluorescent yellow nappy cream on like 'cupcake icing' (their words).

- Other people's baby gear must-have lists. I looked at a lot of these online, and there are some lovely things on them. There are also some truly pointless inventions – wipe warmer, anyone? – and some real overpriced tat. So here is my alternative list: 1) Two really long phone charger cables (2m), so you can read/scroll/message when at the hospital or at home, pinned down by your feeding or sleeping infant; 2) A big plastic bucket for shitty and vomitty clothes; 3) Napisan, a detergent especially designed for poo stains; 4) Bins, not the ones marketed as nappy bins, these are a swizz, just normal bins. The grey ones from Ikea are pretty smell-proof, as long as they are kept out of direct sunlight. (My husband used to sing

'When the sun hits the bin / that we put nappies in / That's appalling' to the tune of 'That's Amore' by Frank Sinatra.); 5) Eye masks and soft silicone earplugs, so you can get some kip if you have a partner who does their shift; 6) Formula, even if you're not planning to use it, in case of any feeding issues; 7) Cook meals for the freezer; 8) Ikea Krama washcloths; 9) Yellow Metanium, the miracle nappy rash cream that they have just discontinued but I hope will have relaunched by the time this book is published, because it was MAGIC; 10) Kindle or clip-on book light so you can read in the dark; 11) Small fire extinguisher, fire blankets, carbon monoxide detector. Look, maybe I'm neurotic, but when you're heating up food while sleep deprived it makes sense to have some bits on hand to keep you and the baby safe.

- The student who fell asleep during our psychological consultation at the NICU. I think he was hungover. While the therapist was busy reassuring us that our bond with our son wouldn't be damaged by his need for medical treatment, and giving us tips on kangaroo care and how to get through this tough time, I noticed that this student's head kept lolling as he struggled to stay awake. I was so focused on my baby that it barely registered, beyond finding it quite funny, but if you had a very sick child, I imagine you'd be livid.

- Without wanting to sound like the observational stand-up bits in *Seinfeld*, the rumours about hospital food were indeed, true. I was overjoyed, however, to discover the South Asian menu on the reverse of the page. Nevertheless, even microwaved daal gets old eventually.

- According to my dad, hand-knitted baby clothes have disappeared from Welsh charity shops, due to trading standards demanding that they need a fire safety label. There used to be such a wonderful range of items, all made by local nains, and though my dad discovered a way to, shall we say, circumnavigate this, it's still a great shame.

- Sleepsuits with poppers that don't match up, sleepsuits with poppers up the back, sleepsuits with no poppers, sleepsuits with weird tie things. As I wrote at the time, they should make them with Velcro so you can simply whip them off, like those satin trousers worn by male strippers. Thankfully, a whole host of readers wrote in with recommendations for alternatives, with Bonds wondersuits being the clear leaders. They have a zip all the way down the front, from the neckline to the ankle, and come in a load of jazzy colours. At around £20 they are on the pricier side, but you can often find them for at least half that on the website BrandAlley, and even cheaper on Vinted and eBay.

- 'The Wheels on the Bus,' the singing of which causes a buried memory to resurface: I was taught – not by my mother – that 'the mummies on the bus go yak, yak, yak,' while the daddies go 'shhh, shhh, shhh.' Unhappy with these retrogressive lyrics, I tried substituting my own. My mummies were 'reading Woolf,' 'taking work calls,' and 'going on a protest,' but if you want to be less pretentious, I quite liked the rhyme time lady's version: 'The mummies and daddies say "I love you".'

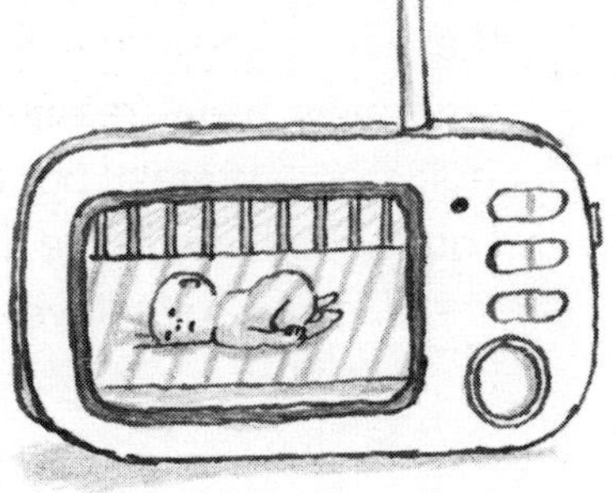

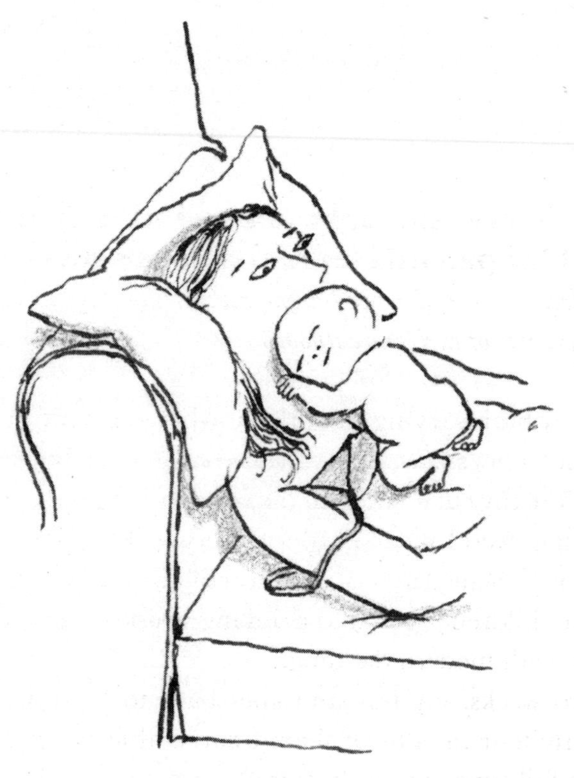

3–6 months

Fathers deserve the right to bond with their babies. Our parental leave system is a mess

(Or: I reflect on the difference having my partner with us made to my experience of early parenthood)

I racked my brains trying to work out what to get my husband for his first Father's Day. A fart-themed mug and a book of dad jokes don't really cut it, after all the weeks and weeks of hands-on fathering. And I mean proper fathering. The Father's Day gift economy, themed as it is around activities that you do away from your children – golf and drinking whisky – hasn't really caught up with modern dadding.

In two weeks, my husband goes back to full-time work, after nearly four months of shared parental leave, and I will become a full-time parent. In this country, most dads go back after the measly two weeks of statutory paternity leave, so our experience is not typical. The culture enables this. My husband has been told socially that there is not much point taking this time, that he won't be able to interact with the baby – who will only be interested in his mother – and will 'just be changing nappies'. No one mentioned bonding.

He has been there, in every sense. He was there in the neonatal intensive care unit with his shirt off, holding the baby against the beat of his heart so that the boy knew from his first hours on this earth that he was loved and protected. He fed me, when I was struggling to feed the child, and sat in on more breastfeeding consultations than anyone should have to. He fed the baby, too, from bottles, right from the beginning, which had not been our plan, but which has only enhanced their closeness and liberated me. He's done the night feeds and the rocking to sleep and the post-jab Calpol. They bowl around the neighbourhood together, the baby strapped to his chest in a way that Piers Morgan would hate. He can make our child smile with the widest, purest grin I've ever seen. And yes, he's had a fair bit of baby shit up his arm, too.

All dads should have this, I think, if they want it. It shouldn't be such an immense privilege to get to bond with your child. In her book *The Life of Dad: The Making of the Modern Father*, Dr Anna Machin says that bonding between father and infant is a two-stage process. The first stage happens at birth, is underpinned by oxytocin, and 'relies upon the biological connection between father and child provided by genetic relatedness'. The second stage comes much later, because 'it is based upon conjoined lives and interactions and is promoted by the much more powerful bonding chemical beta-endorphin, leading to a more profound and much deeper love'. Take the time at the beginning, however, and it feels to me as though the second stage can be reached much more rapidly.

For many dads, the stuff about feeling like a spare part isn't incorrect. If they aren't around full-time for long, they might feel like the secondary parent right from the beginning, 'standing outside … this woman's world', as Kate Bush has it in 'This Woman's Work', her moving and daring song about fatherhood. 'Dads who are thrown back into the office after a couple of weeks never get the chance to bond with their children, which is horrible,' my colleague Alex Hern told me (he took six months to be his daughter's primary caregiver). 'That's the part that is unimaginable to me; it just feels, from the privileged vantage point of not having had to do that, like such an awful thing to inflict on a new parent.

'There's a huge difference between "looking after" your baby and "being in charge of" your baby, and it was crucial for my relationship with my partner for me to have been in charge of my daughter for long enough that I stopped asking how she had done things, and started doing things my way. It means we've come out the other side of leave with an approach to parenting that blends both our experiences.'

This is backed by the research. Sociology professors Paul Hodkinson and Rachel Brooks, whose book *Sharing Care* examines the experiences of fathers who have taken more of an active role in sharing care for their children, conclude that 'the sharing of parental leave from early in babies' lives may make it easier for caregiving fathers to take on full responsibility for emotional and organisational aspects of care later on'. This would help alleviate the disproportionate care burden that continues to fall on women.

Though we've enjoyed shared parental leave, it was unpaid, so we have taken a large financial hit and I've been writing this column throughout. As a policy, it has been a failure, with only 3 to 8 per cent of eligible couples taking it (the UK government has yet to publish the results of its long-promised consultation on this policy). It is still not available to the self-employed.

It's also unnecessarily confusing, and took me a couple of weeks to get my own head around it, simply because it was so poorly explained by most websites. According to a new survey from Pregnant Then Screwed, just half of dads believe their employer understands how shared parental leave works. It breaks down the numerous ways in which men are discouraged from taking the time, from the financial hit (cited by more than half of dads as the reason for not taking shared parental leave) to discrimination in the workplace (16 per cent).

The fact that the shared parental leave policy involves 'taking' leave from your female partner is spectacularly ill-conceived, with women not wanting to relinquish their time and some dads not wanting to 'deprive' their partners of it. As for our pathetic two weeks of paternity leave, 97 per cent of respondents do not believe that two weeks is long enough, and one in four dads say that they continued to work while on paternity leave, with half saying that there was an expectation from their employer that they would, which is unlawful.

Though companies are starting to offer enhanced parental leave to men, if the UK is to catch up with the many other countries that offer properly paid, ring-fenced paternity leave, we need to rip up the shared parental leave policy and start again. This was one of the demands of the Pregnant Then Screwed March of the Mummies, a national protest for parents that took place on 29 October 2022, during which 15,000 families marched in eleven UK cities. The protest's other demands were good quality affordable childcare for all children and flexible working as the default.

If men want more time with their children, they are going to have to fight for it alongside their partners. The key to this, I think, is to start framing paternity leave as crucial bonding time for men and their children, which they are currently being denied. As my husband says, it's been one of the most rewarding times of his life. It should be a right, not a privilege.

I'm learning to live with my fear for my baby's safety: it's the price we pay for love

(Or: How the terror doesn't dwindle, but it does become more manageable as time passes)

I write this from a house that is slowly emerging from Covid, which finally caught us after two and a half years of the pandemic. In some ways, nursing a small, sick baby with a sick husband while also very sick myself was a more hellish experience than childbirth. There were points at which I wondered how we would be able to care for him. Thankfully my mother arrived bearing Calpol and some seriously old-school cough syrup, and for the past week has been feeding us and nursing us, risking her own health in the process.

These challenges mean that I have been thinking rather a lot about fear and how it relates to parenthood. The baby's history of breathing problems meant that I was genuinely frightened when we caught the virus, and though I knew it didn't affect children much, a child I happen to know and love had a very severe reaction to the disease. That, as well as my son's time in a newborn intensive care unit, made it difficult not to let myself become consumed by terror, and yet somehow I coped. While I was there, I saw some very sick babies and some very frightened parents. There was a moment in the bedroom, as I feverishly rocked him back and forth, when I semi-hallucinated all the women who had done the same with their own sick offspring. Most of us need only look at our own family trees to see multiple infant mortalities. In my own family's history is a tale of returning home from burying one child to find another dead.

This all sounds rather dramatic, but I'm convinced these past tragedies are somehow encoded in us. They are, after all, part and parcel of the history of humanity, and in many parts of the world continue to be a living reality. Perhaps it's why the other mothers I speak to admit that they, too, check their babies' breathing in the night. How many times in the last few months have I placed my hand to my son's chest to check that he still lives? It makes sense, though: it is only in the past century that we have been able to have much confidence that our babies will survive, and even then you have myriad terrifying, unpredictable threats: SIDS, meningitis, polio – again.

Fear, my mother says, is the price we pay for love. The fear I feel that something will take my child away from me is so terrible that, like an eclipse, it's better not to look directly at it. And yet I am not an especially neurotic mother and nowhere near as anxious as I thought I might be. My history of PTSD – which at one point manifested as health anxiety – meant I considered parenthood with trepidation. Would I be consumed by fear? Would I transmit that fear on to my baby? But the things we believe will happen do not always come to pass.

Though of course, there are the intrusive thoughts. I am grateful to Anne Enright, whose funny, brilliant book *Making Babies: Stumbling into Motherhood* prepared me in a number of ways for the fear. She writes: 'Once, maybe twice a day, I get an image of terrible violence against the baby. Like a flicker in the corner of my eye, it lasts for a quarter of a second, maybe less. Sometimes it's me who inflicts this violence, sometimes it is someone else. Martin says it is all right – it is just her astonishing vulnerability that works strange things in my head. But I know it is also because I am trapped, not just by her endless needs, but also by the endless, mindless love I have for her. It is important to stay on the right side of a love like this.'

Reading these words meant that, when I first took the baby out in his pram and imagined a car ploughing into us, killing us both, I was prepared for the thought. When you have a baby you become a sort of automatic hazard spotter in a world set with traps. Your mind is engaged in a frequent thought experiment: could this hurt the baby? It has, of course, a purpose: survival. I also liken it to what Edgar Allan Poe called 'the imp of the perverse', that urge to do the thing that is wrong and terrible, to throw yourself off the tall building on which you stand, to laugh during the funeral. 'Wouldn't it be awful?' you think. Such thoughts keep you in check.

Of course, when they are out of control, intrusive thoughts can become problematic. Enright sets herself a limit of two or three a day: 'If I get more than that, then it's off to the doctor for the happy pills.' Chloë Hamilton has written movingly about the barrage of intrusive thoughts that she experienced while suffering from postnatal OCD, and her fear that her baby would be taken away from her. Thankfully she is now better, but, she writes, she would have benefited from being able to open up sooner. 'A simple poster, for example, displayed in the ward toilets, detailing not just where to get help but also how common specific thoughts were, would have helped greatly, encouraging me to open up before my thoughts spiralled once I returned home,' she writes.

As the baby has grown bigger and stronger, my fears for him are not so potent, and it is this message that I would like people who are expecting a child, who are worried about being overwhelmed by anxiety, to carry with them. The terror that something will happen to your baby doesn't dwindle, exactly, but it becomes more manageable as time passes, and I'm told even more so with a second child. Furthermore, the child makes the fear liveable by the simple joy of their presence. As if on cue, my son chose the Covid week to start laughing. And as ever, having support helps. Looking through the living room door at my son sleeping in his bassinet on the floor, my mother on the sofa next to him, I felt that more than ever. She ran to me just as I would run to him, because that is love. Of course there's a price for something as big as that.

Learning to see myself as both a feminist and a carer is a joyful surprise

(Or: On finding freedom and happiness in looking after a baby)

I'm supposed to be writing about joy, but I've just been crying my eyes out. Nothing major, just the physical aftermath of illness, sleep deprivation and a baby whose Celtic roots are manifesting themselves in an extreme hatred of hot weather. The thing I am learning about parenthood is that the lows can feel very low, but they are also transient because the joy, oh my God, the joy! It carries you through.

The cult of motherhood, of course, needs no more cheerleaders. The fact that we are all supposed to be so happy-clappy about childrearing has been the source of much maternal unhappiness and frustration. Several women have confessed to me that they didn't feel that powerful, golden oxytocin high you're supposed to feel after giving birth. Instead, the joy grew and grew as they got to know their babies, but still they felt guilty.

The trouble is, I am happy-clappy. Literally, I am happy and I am clappy, because I know it, as the song I've been singing to him endlessly would have it. The baby is a delight at the moment; having learned to laugh, he is doing these big, wide-mouthed gurgly giggles. When he's not a delight, he's a challenge, but the delight makes the hard parts survivable. It can be hard to feel sorry for yourself for long when a baby is giggling at your silliness.

One of the few things I wasn't told about babies before embarking on this journey was that you are supposed to pump their little legs in a bicycle motion to make the wind come out. That was news to me. I do this while continuously chanting 'pumpy pumpy'. It is silly and ridiculous and admitting this probably means I will never be considered a writer of Serious Intellectual Importance. But I have come to realise that any parent worth their salt can only maintain a very low level of gravitas in the face of a small child who demands to be entertained. I speak 'motherese' now, as linguists call baby talk. It's a term my own mother despises, and she still hasn't forgiven Noam Chomsky and Steven Pinker for giving mothers little credit for a child's language acquisition. But, as I said to my son, because I was changing him while his grandmother and I discussed this: 'They are men, so they would say that, wouldn't they, Mr Poopypants?'

I suppose that's the trade-off you make when you have a child. Some people will cease to take you as seriously, especially if you're a woman, but in exchange you also get to not take yourself so seriously. And there is so much happiness to be found in that. I'm still using my brain (why do I feel the need to say this?) but I have found a new freedom in lightness, too.

I have written before that I could have done with a bit more joy and a lot less fearmongering and negativity during pregnancy. I put this down to an overcorrection of the historical taboo of expressing discontent with the demands of mothering. But I think parents are sometimes circumspect about joy for other reasons, too, especially around people who do not have children but want them. In her 2015 book, *Ongoingness*, Sarah Manguso writes: 'My life felt full before becoming a mother, but I've found that trying to say that I prefer having the baby sounds aggressive. In fact I'd felt affronted, before I was a parent, when parents told me, even in the gentlest terms, that they preferred having their children to not having them.'

When I wanted a baby so much that it felt as though the longing for it would suffocate me, other people's joy could feel like a personal slight. It is a very difficult thing, to want a baby and to not have one. In Claire Lynch's memoir, *Small: On Motherhoods*, she writes of the 'slow agony' of being unable to conceive, 'the stinging blows, the unexpected shock of other people's happiness' and then 'the guilt of getting what you always wanted', followed by a failure to be discreet about her happiness despite promising herself she would.

The other problem is that care work is work. It is some of the hardest work that I have ever done, and I have prior experience, so it was hardly a shock. But it is also love, and with that love comes joy. The two are so tightly bound together that to highlight one is, in the eyes of some, to detract from the other. It's bizarre, because you wouldn't be expected to do any other job for free, even if you love it. Yet to do the work of mothering, and to find joy in it, but to also want recompense for it, and societal support, is often framed as an unreasonable demand – despite our economic reliance on all that unpaid labour. And so the joy gets dampened down, as we make our political demands.

It is only relatively recently that I learned to square the feminist in me with the carer in me. The latter is a role I played for much of my adolescence and, though I have never seen it as unfairly foisted upon me, I never truly appreciated how fulfilling it could be. There is beauty and grace in caring for another person, in tending to their body and their needs. I always saw it in others but I never appreciated it in myself. Now, when my boy is crying and I reach for him and hold him in my arms and see him settle into sleep, I take pleasure and validation in that. And, yes, joy.

For modern mothers, the toxic pull of the 'momfluencer' feels inescapable

(Or: On how I really needed to step away from Instagram)

I recently overheard a conversation between some older women about photographs taken early in motherhood. Several expressed regret that they didn't have more pictures from that time, even though they weren't, they said, looking 'their best'. One woman lamented how she destroyed the photographs of her holding her new baby because she hated her appearance, and said she profoundly regrets this now. It made me sad, speaking as it did to the fact that women feel subject to the external, scrutinising gaze of others, even at such momentous events in our lives.

At least these photos were usually only shared with friends and family; now images like these have a potential audience of millions. I can't imagine anything more exposing than putting such intimate photographs online, but the perfect postpartum photo has become as fetishised on social media as the perfect 'golden hour' between mother and baby (meaning skin to skin contact immediately after the birth) is idealised.

Social media has transformed the way my generation views parenthood, just as women's magazines and TV advertising did for older generations. 'Momfluencer' Instagram accounts – most of them run by white, slim, attractive women with immaculate houses and perfectly dressed children – are in your feed even if you don't follow them. In many ways they hark back to the 1950s, projecting an image of domestic contentment, where mothers and daughters dress the same (called 'twinning') and, having dispensed with work outside the home, embody a 'trad wife' aesthetic (internet trend speak for 'traditional wife').

Other posts instruct you to breastfeed at all cost, promise you the secret to postpartum weight loss, or tell you they can solve your babies' sleep problems. (I set my age to 112, so for a long time the ads I got were for wills and hair dye, but the algorithm seems to have sussed it, either believing me to be a miracle of modern science, or an unusually engaged great-grandparent.)

Other mothers tell me that Instagram has been incredibly destructive to their mental health, and in some cases their physical health. Some hypnobirthing influencers scaremonger about medical intervention to the point where women are refusing the care they need (the same influencers were cited again and again as examples of irresponsible, unscientific, unmedicated birth lobbying). One woman tells me she became obsessed with 'wake windows', an unscientific, rigid approach to baby sleep that is popular on social media, and spent hundreds of pounds on sleep courses. Another tells me 'milestones' became a preoccupation, and she would lie in bed at night comparing her child's motor skills with others'. Fitness is another area rife with toxicity, from babies being used as dumb-bells during couples' workouts ('I feel guilty, ashamed of the fourth biscuit and ultimately flick Instagram off in a huff – resolved to be a spherical unfit mess for the foreseeable,' one mother, Jen Mitchell, tells me), to 'bleak' captions about strengthening babies' abdominal muscles.

Another woman tells me she takes issue with the ubiquitous phrase #makingmemories, and how it 'calls into question all the parents who are screaming into pillows or, like me, vaping in the locked toilet at 10 a.m. just for five minutes of alone time'. The hashtag seems to demand that mothers enjoy this precious time. The same woman tells me that a friend with postnatal depression once spent all night scrolling through motherhood-related posts, 'wishing she had that life, the life where your house was clean and your baby slept. I couldn't believe what she was saying, how could she believe that that was all real?'

As well as carrying the weight of a baby, any mother with a smartphone carries with her a portal into the #blessed lives of others, which serves to highlight – especially in a cost of living crisis where parents are struggling to feed their children – what we do not have. It can be so hard to remember that it's all fake, that we never see the photographs of the cupboard full of junk or the child reprimanded for sticky fingers. The bottle of formula and the antidepressants in the nightstand remain hidden; no one is recording the hours of hair and make-up, the lack of spontaneous joy in a life consisting of curated 'moments'.

My own mother boggles at the sheer amount of information available to us now, in contrast to her era, where you usually had a few second-hand books, at least one of which would end up thrown across the room. How are you supposed to learn to trust your own instincts, she wonders, when you are surrounded by so many opinions?

Of course, social media can provide crucial support, as in the case of groups for those who have experienced baby loss, or accounts that document parenting children with special educational needs. One woman tells me how Instagram helped her identify her postnatal anxiety, when midwives and health visitors spoke only of postnatal depression. Lots love @biglittlefeelings for toddler behaviour tips, the nurse and lactation consultant Lyndsey Hookway, the author Sydney Piercey, and the nutrition and weaning expert Charlotte Stirling-Reed. Many women tell me they've unfollowed some accounts, or deleted the app altogether. A useful question to ask is: 'Does this make me feel better, or worse?' If the answer is worse, unfollow or uninstall.

Earlier this year, a *New Yorker* article looked at the phenomenon of the 'hidden mother' in photographs, from women in the Victorian era covering their faces with fabric to appear inconspicuous in infant portraits, to the modern phenomenon of the mother always being the one behind the camera, absent from the visual narrative of family life, because nobody takes her photo, or she fears she will look ugly. You could argue that 'momfluencers' are taking control of the way motherhood is represented, but that doesn't take into account how backwards the iconography of so many of these images are. Weren't we supposed to resist becoming the angel in the house, rather than smugly show off the wings we've been #gifted?

And then, at the risk of sounding hand-wringing, what of the children whose entire lives are documented without consent? Whose parents spend hours posing, editing, uploading, monitoring responses? What will be the mental health impact of making a child a 'public figure' from the moment they are born? The first 'Mommie Dearest' memoir for the Instagram era cannot be far off.

Some babies sleep well, some don't – beware those selling easy fixes

(Or: How parents are bombarded with rituals and superstitions to get our children sleeping through the night)

I'm not going to tell you whether or not my baby is sleeping. If I say he is and your baby is not, then you will hate me. And if I say that he isn't, I will immediately be bombarded with unsolicited advice, usually for a fee. The shysters are already circling.

Besides, nothing lasts for ever. When the baby was very small and I wondered if he might become 'a good sleeper', other parents delighted in telling me about the four-month sleep regression. Then I found a scientific article claiming it was a myth and decided that if I refused to believe in it, then it would not come for me. I'll let you know how that goes, I could say, but I won't. I'm very tired, but most of all I'm tired of talking and thinking about baby sleep.

I keep reading that in the Western world we are obsessed with getting our babies to sleep through the night, when in fact this is neither natural nor, from a safety perspective, desirable (as poet Louise Glück has it: 'Human beings must be taught to love / silence and darkness'). Thankfully for them, no one has attempted to say this to my face, or to the faces of any of the other new mothers I know, several of whom have not had more than two consecutive hours of sleep for months now. For it is not desirable nor safe to have parents losing their minds from sleep deprivation either.

The cliché that lack of sleep is used as a means of torture is regularly trotted out, but the reality of what it can do to your brain is often skirted over, perhaps because it is simply too eerie, too gothic, too downright creepy to fully contemplate. 'I became prey to daydreams and hallucinations, remembering conversations that had not occurred, glimpsing strange creatures through windows and in corners, a continual buzz of activity in my head both infernal and remote, as if a television had been left on in a next-door room,' says the writer Rachel Cusk.

I think of Sylvia Plath's words 'cow-heavy and floral / In my Victorian nightgown', and remember how I prowled the house in the early weeks in my own Victorian nightgown, looking like Bertha Mason from *Jane Eyre*, and probably as much of a fire hazard. Forget operating heavy machinery, I could barely put one foot in front of the other and wept from exhaustion. The desire for sleep became something visceral and monstrous.

Yet, in the small hours I would sit in the glow of the screen, trying to find the answer to 'baby won't sleep', reading and reading until trying to sleep became pointless, because soon he would be awake again. The insomnia is almost more maddening, the irritating singsong of 'sleep when the baby sleeps' echoing in your ears.

At some point, you become aware that there are different camps when it comes to sleep: the co-sleepers, and the sleep trainers. I judge none of them because I have seen first-hand the effects of long-term sleep deprivation on a person: my autistic brother never slept. How my mother stayed sane, I cannot comprehend. Even now, many years later, she has developed a kind of stamina for baby care and an ability to cat nap that leaves me in awe. Recently I woke after sleeping a sleep of the dead to peer through the living room door at her snoozing on the sofa, my son sleeping peacefully next to her in his bassinet, and felt powerfully and tearfully grateful.

And although the thought of a baby being left alone to cry in the dark makes me feel very sad – one baby book suggested keeping a clean set of sheets next to the crib during sleep training, as the baby would in all likelihood cry until he or she vomited – I understand that sometimes you have to try to save yourself in order to continue being able to parent.

Factionalism helps no one, nor is it new. Previous generations had books by Richard Ferber, Gina Ford and a whole host of others, all saying they would be able to help their babies sleep. Our generation has Instagram sleep consultants with no qualifications to contend with. Trends wax and wane, from cry it out to the shush-pat method. We are told not to feed babies to sleep, to put them down 'drowsy but awake', to live our lives according to regimented nap times. The infant sleep industry in the US alone is apparently worth more than $325 million. A £1,000 crib called the Snoo, which swaddles and rocks your baby to sleep in a way that I can't help but feel is a little dystopian, is the must-have Instagram item (several mothers, friends or friends of friends have said that it does, however, work). We've come a long way from the apocryphal leaving the pram at the bottom of the garden.

As parents, we engage in strange rituals and superstitions about baby sleep. At one stage I was convinced the reason my baby slept was because the mattress of his Ark pram bassinet was made from 100 per cent pure wool. He slept so well in his pram that we would place its bassinet inside the SnüzPod – the bedside crib that allows you to 'co-sleep' safely. Or maybe it was Ewan the Sheep, a pulsating sleep aid with millions of acolytes, or the Mahler I played him in the womb. My mother, meanwhile, used to drive me round north London at 2 a.m. in her nightgown. And then there's the rocking and the singing and the white noise, the pink noise, the brown noise (who knew so many types of noise existed?).

Ultimately, though, I'm not sure what any of it means. Of course there are things you can do, but much of how a baby sleeps seems to be simply internal, inherent. Some do, some don't. But that isn't something you can sell. Or not yet, anyway.

Even in the darkest days of new parenthood, I hold on to the thought that this too shall pass

(Or: Words of comfort for when you're having a really shit time of it)

I write this from a pub garden, where I'm wondering if it would be rude to paint my toenails. Having reached a stage of cabin fever that was verging dangerously close to despair, I followed my mother's advice to buy myself a small treat. In this case, a nail polish in a shade called Cheer Up, Buttercup – without considering that I'd need to somehow find the time to put it on.

Time is something I've never had so little of before – ten minutes to inhale a croissant, a moment to brush my teeth – nor have small snatches of it ever felt in such short supply. None of this is news, of course, but when people talk about parenting being hard perhaps what they are really talking about is how relentless a day feels without a small moment of rest.

With that in mind, I've been asking people what gets them through the worst days. The ones where you're bone tired and both you and the baby are crying. One idea, from a medical professional, was to make sure that you leave the house every day on your own, for a breather. If anyone knows how to achieve this, please let me know.

Wine, people suggest a lot. And it's true that wine helps, though I intensely dislike the 'why mummy drinks/mummy needs gin' culture (you would never have a sign in your kitchen that said: Diazepam: Mummy's Little Helper!). It has to be exactly the correct amount of wine – enough to cheer you up and take the edge off your stress, but not so much (and it really takes very little these days after months of abstinence) that you then end up hungover while trying to entertain a baby, which is the worst way possible to spend a hangover, with the exception of attending mass when you don't speak the language and aren't even Catholic (as I did in 2005).

Then you have food, which I'll admit that I did once use as a way of breaking up the mundanity of my sad little life. I'd think to myself, 'Hmm, might have some cheese on toast later', and dark skies would immediately brighten. Not so any more. Once a source of joy and experimentation, food is now merely fuel, wolfed down lukewarm in a separate room from my husband, who has usually worked hard to feed us, only for me to scarcely remember what I ate.

Social contact, people are big on, too. Which is all very well until you've spent all morning trying to get out to the children's centre only to be told that the class is full. It was a bit bleak watching several other mothers and babies being turned away at the door too, our potential friendships crumbling into dust.

Anyway, you keep trying, because what else is there to do? Other parents tell me that remembering that you'll never have to live that day again helps. Viewing everything as a phase is also useful, and it's true that it does go so quickly, you reflect as you fold up all the newborn clothes to put away or donate, wishing that you hadn't spent so much time in the early days looking at cat memes rather than the adorable, ephemeral neonatal wrinkles that have now vanished from your child's face.

It doesn't feel quick, though, when you are singing 'Ten Green Bottles' at the speed of a funeral lament, just to eke out a few more minutes of sitting down (I also do a very slow, lugubrious version of 'Twinkle Twinkle Little Star', and am available for children's birthday parties).

I do think that, of all the coping mechanisms, writing this column has, in many ways, saved me. I'm so grateful for all the advice and support from readers. It has given me a community. And as one parent said, in response to my question of what gets you through the hardest days: 'Watching the little buggers sleeping. All is forgiven – on both sides.' When I look at my baby peaceful in his crib, I feel intense love, but also gratitude. Not everyone who wants a baby gets that privilege, and remembering that stops you moaning too much.

Saying that, it's several days later and my toenails remain unpainted.

What worked

- Foil emergency camping blankets. My friend Shakes sent me a few of these in a care package, saying that babies love them because they are both shiny and noisy. Our son used to love kicking his as he lay on his back on the baby mat.

- Raphael, the painter. Before we all came down with Covid – a horrible experience that I never wish to repeat – I stole away for a few hours to the National Gallery show. It's worth looking up his paintings of babies (painting babies was not a skill many of his artistic contemporaries ever mastered, as the hilarious website Ugly Renaissance Babies demonstrates). I was deeply moved by his depictions of Madonna and child. It was the *Tempi Madonna*, in particular, that made me tear up; Mary's tender expression as she holds Christ to her face brought to mind the fact that the artist lost his own mother when he was very young.

- Cook Meals. Just after we had our son, our friend bought us a voucher for this range of frozen ready meals, and they saved us in the early months (we still eat them now, when we are feeling lazy or knackered or both). They are tasty and good quality, and we now get the vouchers for friends as new baby gifts.

- Jessica Traynor's poetry collection, *Pit Lullabies*, poems exploring early motherhood, often through lyrical reference to nature and the environment. I particularly liked her 'Metaphysical Breast Milk Poem': 'I clamp you to my breast / where your nip is the pinch / of the universe / squeezing into existence.'

- Captain Calamari, a multicoloured toy squid that seems to hypnotise and amuse all small babies.

What didn't

- Baby swimming. I signed my son up for classes at three months old, which, because he came five weeks early, meant he was more like eight weeks old. I genuinely don't know what the fuck I was thinking; none of the other babies were that small, and I don't know why I decided to make things so difficult for myself. 'You're brave,' another mum said to me in the changing room, while he was screaming at the top of his lungs, and I could tell she thought I was totally mad. We abandoned it after two weeks.

- The weather. We had a heatwave that year and at one point it was so hot that I had to spend days at a time consigned to a dark room, breastfeeding under a fan. Two things helped: some organic rose water decanted into a small spray bottle, to spritz both me and the baby, and a Tupperware container in the fridge containing wet flannels.

- Going out, or indeed doing anything at all, in the evenings. When my son was a newborn, it was easy to take him out for dinner, but then the baby entered a cluster-feeding-and-pooing frenzy in the run up to bedtime that meant all bets were off. What I didn't realise then is how much of baby care is just a phase, and that one day we would get our evenings back. At the time, it felt like it would last for ever.

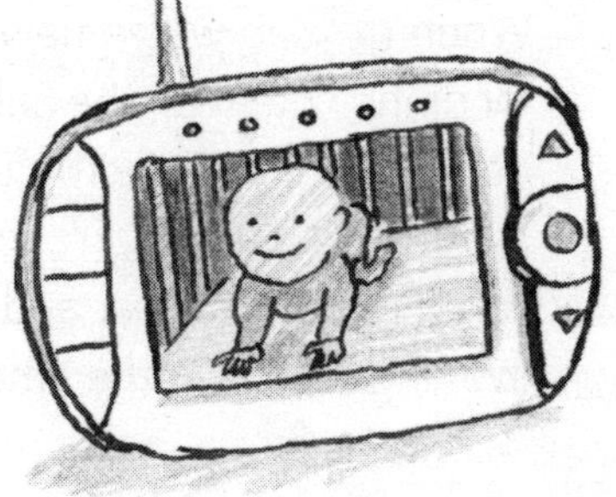

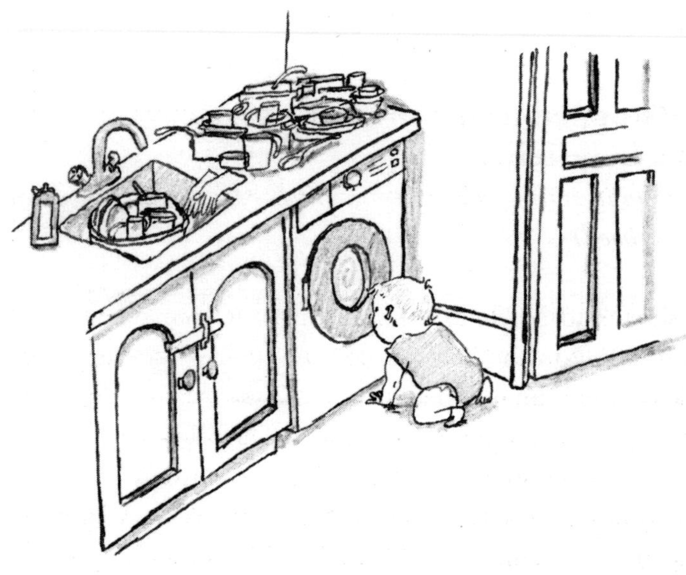

6–9 months

I've stopped trying to be the perfect mum, and it's a huge relief

(Or: On liberating yourself from the sheer insanity of total-reality motherhood)

Flashback to NCT, and I'm asking our course leader Alison about going to the loo: 'So you say that we are not supposed to leave them unattended, ever… so how exactly do I, without putting too fine a point on it… go to the toilet?'

I'm six months in now and have eventually learned that, sometimes, you need to let the baby cry so you can go to the toilet/make a cup of tea/shove a cold samosa in your mouth while you mourn your past life of nicely prepared little lunches. I used to feel guilty doing this. My husband going back to work at four months coincided with the baby suddenly needing constant entertainment, and I started to feel guilty about that too, because sometimes I would put him in the bouncer and read a book (my tight ten-minute set of politically correct nursery rhymes having fallen flat).

Whence had I caught this guilt? Not from my own mother or any of the older women I know. Not social media influencers, whom I avoid completely. And not parenting books, either – I opened *The Wonder Weeks,* observed its literal checklist of developmental milestones, and decided it was a recipe for madness. I had already missed the boat on tummy time.

Research led me to resolve that I had somehow absorbed what Judith Warner calls 'total-reality motherhood'. In other words, it's the cultural notion that motherhood is supposed to constitute your entire life's work, with all other aspects of your identity sacrificed on the altar of 360-degree parenting. It seems this pernicious ideology began in the 1990s but reached fever pitch at the turn of the millennium. These days it afflicts my generation through bastardised, social-media-filtered versions of attachment theory and gentle parenting philosophies. To quote one article: 'Now mothers were always to be "on", engaged in relationships with their children that were at once kinesthetic, tirelessly management oriented, and unrelenting in their emotional solicitations.'

Eliane Glaser frames it as the cult of the perfect mother, elsewhere it's 'intensive mothering' or 'conscientious cultivation'. However it is described, it boils down to the belief that every moment must have conspicuous educational or emotional value. As far as I've read, it is a largely Western construct and is not only bad for women, but also bad for children, who should be allowed to discover the world for themselves or through play with other children. It manifests in the competitive obsession with baby classes, where everything is a learning opportunity (see also the baby sensory movement). Hence, perhaps, my (in hindsight) insane decision to take a three-month-old premature infant to baby swimming, an activity to which he objected to in the strongest terms. What was I thinking? And why did I feel so guilty when we quit?

Perhaps it's all a symptom of highly educated women being stripped of their identities overnight and needing some sort of outlet. Was this why all the other mothers in the introducing-solids workshop seemed to have a professorial knowledge? I started to feel bad until I remembered that I have been consuming solid food myself for many years now with no problems. If I'm still cutting up his food when he's thirty-five, I'll devote some time to feeling bad about doing purees.

I haven't liberated myself from all maternal guilt – that would be impossible – but in the last two months I have been mindfully giving less of a toss and am far happier. The baby is happier too, because his mother is less anxious. None of these proponents of total-reality motherhood ever seem to take maternal mental health into account. Whether it's pushing breastfeeding at all costs or telling you that any kind of sleep training will result in the same sad neglectful hush observed in Romanian orphanages, there never, ever seems to be an acknowledgment that a mother on the verge of a breakdown might do more damage to her kid than a bottle of formula or a short time spent learning to self-settle.

If you're wondering how I managed to successfully purge myself of perfectionism, the answer is that I read two things. First, a research paper by David F. Landy called 'Accounting for Variability in Mother–Child Play' on how mother–child play is culturally and class specific, and actually not always desirable. Second, the book *French Children Don't Throw Food* by Pamela Druckerman, which is a decade old, but totally liberating. Reading it, all of my memories of nannying in France began to resurface, and something clicked into place.

French women are practically unique in the West in that they don't buy this intense perfectionism. They don't ditch their jobs to do childcare, they don't pounce the minute their child needs something, they don't obsess about milestones, and they don't constantly narrate their play (their babies also, apparently, tend to sleep). Most importantly they often – and it feels shocking to even write this – put themselves first.

As Élisabeth Badinter writes in *The Conflict*: 'French women have avoided the dilemma of all-or-nothing motherhood', because 'unlike most Europeans, they have the benefit of historic recognition of their identities beyond motherhood'. Badinter also notes that the childcare system there supports the expectation that the state should provide this service in order to facilitate part-time mothering.

Unfortunately, our own childcare system is sorely lacking – but there is still much to take from the French mindset. I genuinely think Druckerman has saved my sanity. Now, time to feed the baby. But first, I'll feed myself.

Loneliness is a struggle for new parents – can we all stop pretending everything's OK?

(Or: Why it's hard to form friendships with people who just want to talk about mashed avocado)

I experienced a moment of pure, unadulterated joy this week. In St Pancras Old churchyard, watching my son discover a blustery autumn morning for the first time, the wind in the trees causing him to wiggle his head and smile his wide gummy smile, I felt the magic of childhood again, a feeling I thought I'd lost for ever. It was just he and I, together, discovering the world, and for a few minutes it seemed as though I'd never feel lonely again.

Parenthood involves a mix of emotional highs and lows. For every moment like this, there has also been a contrasting one – standing in a different park and feeling an almost physical loneliness. As a writer, I am used to spending many hours happily alone, but for some reason there's nothing like the company of a small child to underscore a feeling of solitude. A study by the British Red Cross found that more than eight in ten mothers (83 per cent) under the age of thirty had feelings of loneliness some of the time, while 43 per cent said they felt lonely all the time. Another survey found that 90 per cent of new mothers felt lonely since giving birth, with over half (54 per cent) feeling they had no friends.

The process of becoming a mother – matrescence, as it's increasingly known – involves huge hormonal changes and a major shift in identity, as well as the uprooting of our usual support structures and routines. This is why, we are told, having 'mum friends' who are experiencing these same changes is so important, and those relationships, between both mothers and their respective babies, can last for life. But cuts to services mean free support groups are harder to find in many areas, and prenatal courses such as those delivered by the NCT can be expensive for people on low incomes. And just because you share one life experience doesn't mean that you'll have much else in common (which is one reason why I think it's so important to keep spending time with your child-free friends and not abandon them, as some do). Sometimes other mothers can be standoffish and competitive, or simply too exhausted to engage beyond a few polite hellos. Women who have migrated here also face linguistic and cultural barriers, as well as being separated from their own family networks, exacerbating their potential social isolation.

In a recent interview, the comedian and writer Daisy May Cooper spoke of how hard she found it to befriend other mothers when she had her baby. 'If I see your vulnerability, then I'm there, like a moth to a flame,' she said. 'But I've never been able to connect with, for example, the women that I met in my neonatal group who were trying to pretend everything was all right. And you'd go, "Come on, let's have a glass of wine, tell me what's really going on." "Oh no, everything's fine! Let's just talk about the kids!" The WhatsApp group was just thousands and thousands of messages about mashing up avocados. I thought, if I can't penetrate that surface then I'm out, I'm just not interested.'

I agree. I'm more interested in befriending the women to whom you can complain about your bruised breasts or who tell you how much they miss smoking a joint in the bath, than the ones who – as brilliantly satirised in the Australian comedy *The Letdown*, which revolves around an antenatal group – eye your coffee suspiciously and say: 'Not breastfeeding, then?' Thankfully I've only met a couple of judgy types, one of whom asked me what my baby's birth had been like as an opening gambit and followed it up with a pass-agg 'never mind, he's here now' before telling me all about her own birthing-pool floating, carrot-juice drinking, house-music listening experience.

I've been incredibly lucky that the women I have met and befriended in neonatal groups have been frank and funny about the challenges of motherhood, and a WhatsApp group of university friends with young children provides crucial moral support. When I was pregnant, I joined Peanut, a social networking app that aims to connect pregnant women, but I was almost instantly put off by the girlboss 'you've-got-this-babe tone' of the Q&A profile prompts ('You're a woman! You're already a superhero!' 'If an actress would play me it would be… Jennifer Aniston'). A friend that I met at a free parenting group run by the council recently mentioned that she'd messaged me and I'd not responded, so perhaps I should have given it more of a chance. As for Mumsnet, Daisy May Cooper's darkly funny *Am I Being Unreasonable?* is named after the website's famous discussion board, to which she was addicted when her marriage was falling apart. The site doesn't feel aimed at my demographic (and like any social media platform it has its proportion of unhinged members), but it provides many women with a vital support system at a vulnerable time in the same way that previous generations had the National Women's Register or Sure Start.

We know that, for new mothers, loneliness can exacerbate postnatal depression – just one reason why Conservative cuts to Sure Start are such a desperately sad scandal. Living in Islington, which has retained early-years centres under the 'Bright Start' banner, has been a privilege because of the sheer range of groups and activities available to parents free of charge. All parents should have access to these services (postnatal depression and loneliness affects dads, too). Sadly, little has changed on this front, but at least there are small comforts – the friendliness of strangers has been amazing to me. Every day, someone reaches out to me and my son with a kind word, a smile or a question. Perhaps they have been there themselves, and are paying it forward, as I will, too, if I see a new mum or dad at the playground, looking lonely or lost.

I hated being told I should 'cherish every moment' of motherhood – now I understand

(Or: In which I take the time to remember)

Of all the phrases parents tell me they dislike, 'cherish every moment' is the winner. Time is a strange thing when you are caring for small humans, and, as I thought about it this week, it is this phrase that keeps coming back to me. It's the idea that by feeling any negative emotion, you are somehow squandering time. I have been told by parents with postnatal mental health issues that this unrealistic phrase – often said by older people – has made them feel deep shame. Time is precious, and to not feel constantly delighted by your child is a terrible waste.

I don't feel shame, but I'll confess that the occasional suggestion that this column is overly negative has wounded me. I've been writing it in real time these past eight months – I wrote notes for my first column while in hospital, the sounds of women in labour all around me – and though there have been struggles, there have also been immense, intense highs. My son still feels miraculous to me. But writing as it happens means real, living feelings land on the page, some dark, some light. There's no time to try to temper reality in retrospect to make it seem like it's always plain sailing.

When I see new parents out and about with newborns, I feel solidarity but also a strange mix of other emotions. He was once so small and curled like a bug – how could that time have passed so quickly? Why did I not realise how short those days would be? At the time they felt unceasing; in the whirl of feed, sleep, feed, sleep I could not see an end to them. The baby and I were still one, and would cease to be. He would open his eyes to the world and look beyond me, and I would be gifted a whole new phase, while mourning that which came before. At the time, the shock of his premature arrival left little room for reflection – but had you asked me, I'd have maybe said that I felt that the time in the third trimester, when the baby should have still been safe inside me, had been lost, or even stolen. Now I say I got five extra weeks of him. What a gift, this time travel.

When you are raising a child, it isn't that the hard parts aren't hard, but that time marches on so indefatigably that they almost mystically fade. Older people, I think, understand this, which is why they often can't remember when you ask them about specific aspects of parenting, such as my mum not recalling when she moved on from giving me purees, or how they coped with certain difficulties. (In case it sounds as though her memory is going, she just recited T. S. Eliot to the baby: 'I have measured out my life with coffee spoons.' I could measure the last year of mine in formula scoops, I thought.)

Women have said to me that they suspect this amnesia might be evolutionary, otherwise no one would have a second child. Time makes you sentimental, and pain fades in the memory, with sleeplessness rendering whole stages – where the passing of time felt like treacle – a blur. I'm starting to understand that. The hell of establishing breastfeeding felt, at the time, all consuming. I doubt I'll ever fully forget it, but thinking about it now is like watching a film about someone else, while sitting a great distance from the screen.

Older people also give you outdated advice, like telling you to start babies on solids at four months. That's the other thing about time: the official recommendations around parenting change so often that sometimes older generations might be made to feel that their input is irrelevant. This is not the case. The science around safe sleeping may be different, but my mother still knows, it seems, instinctively how to comfort and entertain a baby, and I am tearfully grateful for her years of graft and wisdom. The letters I've had from older readers that say this series brings it all back to them vividly have been some of the most moving to me.

Of course, you can let time get on top of you if you allow it to. On a tough day, you can find yourself staring down the barrel of the next eighteen years, wondering if you've got what it takes. But then you find yourself excited about showing the baby *The Wizard of Oz* for the first time – and of all the joys to come.

The other thing about time is that it becomes a precious commodity: time to yourself, time to work, time to think. My husband and I are constantly trying to find time. When he isn't working, he's with the baby, trying to give me a break. Meanwhile, I'm working while the baby sleeps. Should I be watching the flutter of his long eyelashes, his cupid's-bow mouth slightly opened, instead? I wonder. He will only be this exact way once, and I'll have missed it typing this.

And so I put down this column, and I take a minute or five to gaze at him, and stroke the fine tuft of his hair. I may not cherish every moment – some of the nappies I have changed render that impossible – but I am taking a little time every day to look and to feel and to try to remember, to set it all in amber: the sound of his breath, the curve of his head, his smell, his fat little fingers curled around mine. Perhaps this – finding moments to cherish – is what those well-meaning people mean.

I don't know where the time goes, but I know that one day I'll be glad I wrote it down.

There is nothing like a trip to A&E with a sick baby to make you eternally grateful for our NHS

(Or: Fuck bronchiolitis)*

It's when the nurse in the triage room says, 'I'll just finish filling this form in later,' that my blood turns to ice. I always thought that expression was a cliché, but in that moment it became true, and I entered a full-body state of panic. The baby, on the other hand, is pale and smiling, almost serene despite having been yanked from sleep and rushed up the road. But his readings, clearly, are not good.

Other parents tell me that these trips to A&E are a rite of passage. We have been to A&E four times since the baby was born. This is our second trip today. This morning, he was on the borderline for admission, so I know what he has – bronchiolitis – and that he'll need oxygen. What I don't know is how bad it may get. No one knows that. Some babies recover quickly, I'm told, and some can become seriously unwell. The medical staff are calm and reassuring, but they are setting up the equipment, taking the infant-sized oxygen mask out of its packaging, and attaching the monitor to the baby's toe, with ominous speed.

The baby had gone to sleep this evening, and I was about to join him. But a niggling fear made me send a video of his breathing to my aunt Jane, a retired GP. 'You'll need to get him checked again,' she said. I am so grateful for her now, thinking that I could have been at home asleep as he deteriorated next to me.

'He's not going to die,' the nurse says to me, when I ask her.

---

* My editor Kirsty and I joked at the time that this should have been the headline on the piece.

She brings me a cup of tea. The computer screensaver says the hospital is in category four, a 'major incident'. They've found a bed for us in a room at the back. When they say they need to try high-flow oxygen and will put a feeding tube in at the same time, I have to leave the room to be sick.

I feel bad for all the parents in the waiting room who have to listen to me from the toilet next door, whose kids are lying across their laps or on seats, some of them stripped off to help their fevers. The NHS is crumbling from deliberate underfunding but we have been lucky enough to be seen in under five minutes. This morning, I heard a nurse tell a colleague who arrived for their shift, 'I'm not going, I can't go.' Later, I hear a doctor mention that she hasn't had lunch.

I feel profoundly grateful to the staff as they hook my baby son up to the machines. I am impressed, as I always am when observing medical staff. What a thing, to know how to do this. And to treat us with such kindness, and such patience, when the oxygen tube dislodges yet again and we ask them to come and reposition it for the fourth, fifth, eighteenth time.

This year, the NHS helped my son into the world, and it helped nurse a dear friend to her death. That is its mission, from cradle to grave. I agree with the American writer and comedian Rob Delaney that it is the pinnacle of human achievement.

They didn't need the feeding tube in the end. At 2 a.m., the baby feeds from me for forty-five minutes, and I cry, deliriously tired, with relief. He seems to be gaining strength. By late morning, when we are moved to the children's ward, they say he could be home by the evening. One of the nurses jokes that it's because I went home and brought back so much stuff. 'If you hadn't, we'd be keeping you in, it's always the way.' She spends all winter looking after babies with bronchiolitis. Thank you, I keep saying, thank you, thank you, thank you.

At home, the adrenaline is dwindling, and I am left shaken and tired. I feel very lucky, and maybe a little bit silly as the baby's illness is not uncommon. I feel as though we've joined the ranks: all those pale, ghostlike parents who carried their children towards the bright glow of A&E, who also spent last weekend on camp beds and plastic chairs, hoping their kids would be OK. Some will be home already and some will only be at the start of their medical journey. Some, and I can barely think of this, won't have survived. All of us will have used the NHS. It hangs by a thread, but its heart is still beating.

Why is my baby crying? I used to google for hours – then discovered the real answer

(Or: On how the internet is killing parental instinct – and maybe the baby boomers had it right)

The longer I spend as a parent, the more I realise that it's a bit like being a detective, and not only because I look strung out, wear a trench coat and am full of droll maxims such as: 'You can have a hangover from other things than alcohol. I had one from a baby.'

Having a baby who can't tell you what's going on with it means having to solve a mystery every single day. Say the baby is whingeing: first, you run through the usual checklist. Is the baby hungry? Is his nappy full? Is he sleepy? Does he have wind? Once you've ascertained which one it is, you go back to the start, because it's probably something else by now.

There are deeper mysteries, of course, than this. When I realised my baby was waking up because his hands were getting cold, it was via a process of elimination that took several weeks. But that didn't stop well-meaning readers from trying to crack the code. I think as humans we have an instinct towards problem-solving, and more experienced parents can well recall the hours they spent trying to work out the reasons why their baby was doing this or that. Sometimes my mother, my husband and I will all find ourselves speculating together in the living room in an exhausted summit. Could it be teeth? The change in the seasons? All that adult brainpower dedicated to one tiny infant.

Your baby is probably hungry, one correspondent informed me – and I mean no ill will towards him, because he is a doctor and a parent, and more experienced than I. In this case he was wrong, though his recommendation of putting butter in the puree to keep the baby fuller for longer was helpful for an entirely different reason, in that broccoli tastes better with butter. We know this as adults, yet somehow expect our babies to accept naked vegetables from the off.

I suppose what I'm saying is that, even if the reader's suggestion isn't the answer at that moment, it could well be the answer further down the line, or indeed the key to an altogether different mystery. So I'm grateful to all the amateur sleuths out there for doing some of my work for me.

It's when you bring the whole internet into it that it becomes problematic, as I learned during one of my late-night Google sessions when the baby went through a phase of waking forty-five minutes after being put down at bedtime, which I learned is called a 'false start'. The reasons listed were as follows: too many naps, not enough naps, overtired, undertired, wake windows, hunger, allergies or separation anxiety.

Not a single one of the reasons listed was wind. So, even though each time I picked the baby up he would do the kind of almighty burp that you usually hear from an adult man doing his best Barney Gumble impression, I did not trust my instincts. The same thing happened when all the websites said that teething doesn't disrupt sleep. I believed them, got myself into a stress about why the baby wouldn't settle, ignored the gnawing pain every time I fed him, and then, lo and behold: a fang appears, waving a big flag that reads 'idiot'.

There is simply too much information out there. Too many people with agendas and opinions. Why would a thread of Mumsnet users know the reason for your baby's rash? Of course, I love the internet. The internet means that you can make a quick exit from your local art house cinema, where your child has been loudly farting through Kazuo Ishiguro's exquisite screenwriting, in order to google, 'What the hell is that in my baby's nappy?' and get the response, 'Don't worry, they just had banana!' in a fraction of a second.

In the olden days, you would have had to go to a payphone to phone your mother, and she probably would have been out drinking a snowball at a cocktail party and eating savoury jelly, so you'd have had to go to the library and look it up. Or else maybe you'd have shrugged your shoulders and thought: 'Eh. It'll probably be OK.'

But the internet is also killing parental instinct. Millennials are so used to being able to instantly receive the answer to any minuscule bit of trivia that when we can't solve a mystery such as why our baby is crying, it drives us insane. I've found that one solution is to channel our boomer predecessors by not worrying so much and hoping for the best. One friend seems to have successfully managed this – it helps, I think, that she has two, and all the wisdom that goes with that. 'I just accept that some days he will cry all day and some days he will be cheery, just like some days I wake up in a bitch of a mood,' she says.

So why waste the energy? With the exception of illness, a grumpy baby is par for the course, and rarely a great mystery that needs solving. Nowt lasts for ever, as my mum says. In any case, it's probably wind.

Grandparents are the invisible glue, holding our broken childcare system together

(Or: On being grateful for your parents, while wishing they didn't have to give so much)

I bought a book for my mother and the baby to read together. *I Love My Granny* talks about her 'comfy tummy' and the fact that she has 'lived for ages' and has 'loads of time' on her hands, which frankly I find a bit rude. Nevertheless, it speaks to the loving and caring role that a grandparent can have in a child's life. Seeing my baby bond with his grandparents has been one of the most rewarding aspects of being a parent so far.

The UK's broken childcare system means that grandparents often have to step in to offer help, with one study finding that 85 per cent offer some kind of support when it comes to looking after grandchildren. My parents are no different – my mum especially has been very present these past months – while my dad and stepmum, the baby's *nain* and *taid* (Welsh words for grandmother and grandfather), practically begged to take him so we could swim in the sea and go out for dinner. His paternal grandparents have cared for his many cousins who live locally to them.

I must say I'm relieved that the baby has finally got a nursery place, as I've been feeling guilty about the amount of childcare my newly retired mum has been helping us with. I'm incredibly grateful and I've treated her to a posh spa day to mark her retirement and to say thank you, as well as covering her trains (she lives up north). She adores the baby and loves being with him, and he loves his 'nonna', so it's not all toil. Nevertheless, it doesn't feel great that after decades of caring for my brother, who is autistic, and me, she is now taking on more labour just as she should be able to relax. I also feel guilty that she has been spending nights on the sofa, and that she caught Covid from us when she came to help. I owe her a great debt for sharing her time, wisdom and experience with my new little family.

I'm not the only one who feels guilty. One mother of a one-year-old tells me she has had to draft her mum in two days a week due to a lack of nursery spaces. It was that, she says, or resign. 'I feel so guilty about the whole situation, even though it's not really my fault,' she writes. 'It's such a burden on my mum – she is relatively young but it's not fair to take up so much of her time with the slog of everyday childcare rather than her being able to savour special moments with my daughter at her convenience and leisure. It goes without saying that my mum is doing this all unpaid and wouldn't accept it if we offered. To be honest, the fact that it is unpaid also means we can actually afford for me to be at work.'

Of course, there's a difference between gratefully, and guiltily, accepting freely given offers of help and feeling entitled to it. One of the most bemusing aspects of the comedy series *Motherland* is the level of entitlement that stressed mum Julia, the protagonist, feels towards her mother, not to mention her mother's indifference to her grandchildren. Furthermore, the close parent–child–grandchild relationships that many of us treasure are not everyone's experience, and geography is a huge factor.

And what of grandfathers? It's largely grandmothers who do the bulk of the caring, and I wonder if the sense of entitlement some parents feel to their labour can be blamed on tradition. Throughout human history, grandmothers played a large role in the upbringing of children, especially in working-class families where the mother was needed for paid work outside the home. Can we blame some of our mothers' generation of second-wave feminists for resisting that, or for wondering when exactly the hard, physically demanding work will stop?

There are, of course, hands-on grandfathers (my dad is one, a man comfortable with all aspects of childcare). 'My dad and I joke that he's the world's best grandpa, or an average grandma,' another mum, who has a three-year-old autistic son and a young baby, tells me. 'My mum passed away years before I had children and my in-laws live further away, so I am very grateful he's stepped up, and the relationship he has with his grandson is so beautiful.' Her son's autism has made childcare difficult so her dad does two afternoons a week. 'My dad's always been good with toddlers and babies. He's great at story time, can really make them laugh and talks to them like little adults, which they always appreciate,' she says. 'But he wasn't much for practical stuff, he didn't really change nappies for me and my siblings when we were babies and hadn't changed any for my son until we discussed the idea of him helping out when I went back to work.'

As well as all the hands-on help, it's lovely to read about the joy that grandchildren can bring to their grandparents. Take this recent comment beneath my column, from a grandfather: 'I have largely brought up my granddaughter from the age of less than a week. In my 80s, I am quite capable of changing nappies, feeding, wiping up enormous messes, dealing with all the tantrums and tears. It's a privilege. It always was. At my age, I will never dance at her wedding, so I dance with her now.'

What worked

- The Babyzen YoYo pram. I loved our Ark pushchair with bassinet and we still use it, but as we transitioned to a sitting position and the baby gained more and more weight, it made sense to have a lighter option, too. There's a reason that everyone in north London has this stroller: it's light, it's compact, it fits in an overhead compartment when you're travelling, and I found it totally liberating, as all the best design is.

- Baby's first newspaper. It's a crinkly sensory cloth book called *The Nursery Times*, and all of the stories are about dinosaurs, but you have to start somewhere.

- 'All I Have to Do is Dream' by the Everly Brothers. My mum started singing this to him and he loved it so much that I started playing it on my phone, which I would place in the bassinet of the pram as I pounded the pavements of north London. Being unable to access my device while doing this made me start fantasising about a pram with built-in Bluetooth speakers.

- The children's classic *Peepo!* A few years ago, the archaeologist Gabriel Moshenska tweeted that the book is rooted in the material culture of the Second World War, and I enjoyed noting the references on every page: a gas mask, a ration book, a portrait of Churchill.

- Ashton & Parsons teething gel. On top of illness, these were the months of endless teething, and this gel – which was recommended by many, many parents – seemed to do the trick.

- *Hushabye Lullabye*. We didn't adhere to the 'no telly until eighteen months' recommendation. After my son was hospitalised, we were encouraged to avoid infection for a while and therefore to steer clear of baby classes, cafes, etc. I tried to keep him occupied with books and singing but every now and again I would put this on, which is colourful, gentle and soothing. I still feel obscenely grateful to Sacha Kyle, the creator of this televisual equivalent of temazepam.

- Prune puree. If you need to ask why, then I envy you (too much Greek yoghurt was the culprit).

What didn't

- Baby-led weaning (BLW). I found the pressure to give the baby big chunks of food to play with – as per current fashionable orthodoxy – rather intense. One woman, a stranger, even came up to us in the pub and told us we should be doing it. Lots of parents, mothers especially, placed a moral value on it in a way I found bizarre. In hindsight, I think the extent to which I was worried about him choking was probably a sign I hadn't fully processed the birth yet, but I trusted my instincts and stuck to purees until I felt he was ready, and, contrary to what I was told, he has become the opposite of a picky eater.

- Having to book baby classes in advance. It cost me a fortune that virus-ridden winter, when we were constantly missing classes we had already paid for.

- Me. I started finding it very hard to write at home, where I could often hear the baby crying from the living room. In the first year, the cry of your own child feels visceral and is almost impossible to ignore, so I was constantly having to go through to feed him. My mum was around a lot that autumn and winter and so would take him out in the pram, but I did end up having to dictate my column to her on at least one occasion. I was beginning to realise that I had been quite naive about how I would juggle both.

- Having an indoor cat – Mackerel's choice, not ours – and a baby in one flat proved rather challenging. I trod barefoot in cat sick while changing a nappy, and it wouldn't be the last time.

- The car. My son hated his car seat, so taking taxis was a nightmare, despite the best efforts of some lovely Uber drivers, one of whom blasted 'Twinkle, Twinkle Little Star' through the car speakers to calm him. I decided to start taking the bus more – until he got sick, that is. So much of parenthood is a steep learning curve. I couldn't, for instance, work out how to get off the bus without the pram tipping towards the gutter, and it wasn't until a friend pointed out that you're better off doing it backwards that I was able to achieve this with any poise.

- Socialising. Two hospital stays in less than a month meant jettisoning plans in an attempt to help the baby recover.

- Sleep. Illness, teething and separation anxiety meant that during this period the baby went from being a good sleeper to waking every hour. He stopped wanting to sleep on his back in his crib altogether. We started co-sleeping, though that meant he started waking throughout the night to feed. I felt proud of being able to nurse him through nasty virus after nasty virus, and cherished our closeness, but at times I felt that I was on the verge of losing my mind.

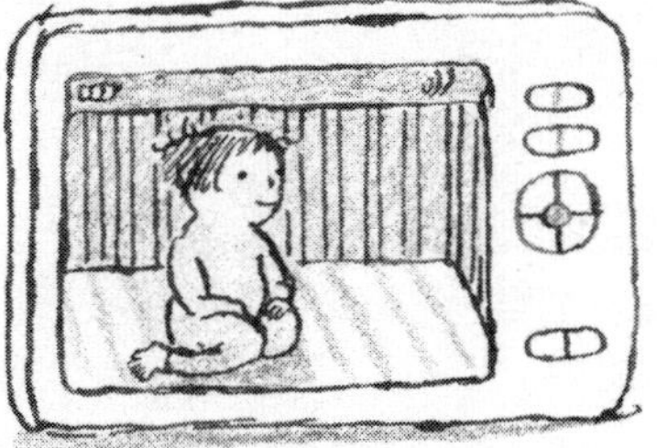

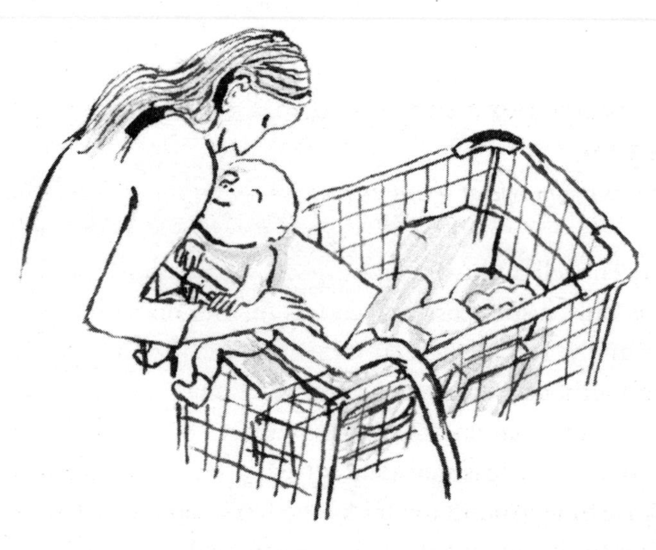

9–12 months

I've always felt a tug of sadness at Christmas – until this year

(Or: On the magic of seeing the festive season through a baby's eyes)

I've been well and truly ambushed by Christmas this year: the tree is only just decorated, and as for the home-made wreath I normally lovingly create with greenery foraged from the neighbourhood – forget it. I'm late on everything, from sending my tax information to my accountant to this column. I've missed all the Christmas delivery windows, and have spent this week rushing around town like the harassed mother I now am. Owing to illness and the baby forgetting how to sleep without the breast, I have missed every single festive gathering, both personal and professional, including the Guardian Opinion do, a huge family weekend in a Welsh haunted house, and various literary events, the schmoozing element of which could well have helped the chances of my new book – reference to which I have shoehorned in here in the hope that it might drum up some preorders. I have drunk precisely one (one!) martini, my first in eighteen months, and while I enjoyed it, I would rather have had three, despite everyone knowing that two is the tipping point.

Yet I couldn't be happier. Despite the opening paragraph, if you've come here for a protracted whinge, you will go away disappointed. This mad, chaotic singular year, I have felt the meaning of Christmas more than perhaps any other. I am the very essence of joy to the world, peace on earth, good tidings etc., etc. I haven't even touched my misanthropic Merry Fucking Christmas Spotify playlist, because I don't wish I had a river I could skate away on. I'm happy right here, with my husband and my baby, and though I may roll my eyes during lullaby time when I get to lines such as 'holy infant so tender and mild' and 'the little Lord Jesus no crying he makes' it is only momentary. This year, I have had a great gift bestowed upon me, the gift of a child, and it has changed everything.

It's not as though I hated Christmas before. I was no Scrooge; I got into the spirit, but I was always acutely aware of the melancholic side to the season, a festival of feasting and light in a darkness that is never entirely absent despite our best efforts, as we think of loved ones we have lost and Christmases past and feel, or I do anyway, a tug of sadness at the fact that we will never live those innocent childhood memories again. Divorce, bereavement, illness, poverty, pain – all families face challenges, and Christmas can have a tendency to cast them in high relief.

In my case, being a child of divorce with a brother in a care home, it was the scattered nature of my family, so different in its patterns and traditions from the wholesome, conventional groupings we see in adverts, and the stress of travelling from pillar to post to be with everyone I loved in a short window of time, that sometimes made me feel less than jolly. Perhaps this is why my favourite carol is 'In the Bleak Midwinter' and my favourite Yuletide song is 'Christmas Card from a Hooker in Minneapolis'. I took a morose joy in the defiant and the non-traditional, the saturnine and the grinchy, the ghostly and the uncomfortable. The darkness at the edge of the toy town.

While it is true that I will never experience a childhood Christmas again – will never fully live the excitement of my first real tree in its red bucket, with its hot, multicoloured twinkle lights enclosed in little plastic petals, or the anticipation of leaving a wee dram for Santa on the fireplace before heading to bed – I feel that I have been gifted something greater. Because I get to see it through the eyes of my baby son, and I get to devote my time to giving him his first Christmas. From taking him to get the tree, to describing the decorations as he watches me decorate it, singing carols to him, and seeing his face as he watches the lovely *Mr Bear's Christmas* on CBeebies (narrated by Stephen Fry, it's an eleven-minute DIY animation by the self-published author Lorna Gibson, crafted from felt, wool and foam and shot on an iPhone using a £5 stop-motion app), it's all been magical so far. I've loved dressing him in a Christmas jumper, charity shopping for toys and choosing the books that will become his favourites.

Most special of all, however, was our trip to see the lights at Kenwood House earlier this month. We went last year, when I was pregnant with him, my stomach swelling, my walk on its way to becoming a waddle, my fears about Covid and the prospect of giving birth in an understaffed maternity unit frightening me more than I let on as I posed next to the tree. To return with him bursting with excitement at the lights as snowflakes kissed his red, cold cheeks and he kicked his legs as his dad carried him in the sling was one of the best moments of my motherhood so far. Seeing a dad chase his toddler, who had illegally broken into a light installation and was running around, gave me a glimpse of what my life will look like next year. The next morning, I watched my son shake the snow that had fallen overnight from the branches in the garden.

This time of year can be tough for lots of reasons. I'm not suggesting that having a baby can melt it all away, but it does feel as if I've undergone a personal shift. Instead of being haunted by the ghost of Christmas past, I'm embracing the ghost of Christmas future. It's all for him now. All of it.

I left my baby to write this. How do artists balance creativity and the ache for their child?

(Or: The fire is still on, I'm just on the back burner)

Since having a baby, I have never felt more creatively inspired, and never more frustrated. 'The fire is still on, I'm just on the back burner,' I might say – one of the phrases in the artist Andi Galdi Vinko's transcendent photo book, *Sorry I Gave Birth I Disappeared But Now I'm Back*.

It chronicles motherhood in all its strange, visceral, leaky realism, as well as its naturalistic beauty. Recently, it has become a visual bible for me, as I wonder what it is to be on the back burner, or even to disappear, at a time when the tension between caring and creating has never felt more acute.

In order to do both, you have to, it seems, put the proverbial baby on the fire escape. It's probably apocryphal, but this is what the painter Alice Neel's in-laws claimed she did in order to work. I've been savouring the book, *The Baby on the Fire Escape: Creativity, Motherhood and the Mind–Baby Problem*, these past months. It looks at how celebrated female artists and writers, such as Neel, Doris Lessing, Alice Walker and Ursula K. Le Guin navigated the demands of motherhood into the need to create. The author Julie Phillips tried to find a common thread between how these women made it work, but instead was confronted with 'a negative space, an impossible position'.

Whether it is relying on a network of 'othermothers' for support, having a partner who does their share or more of the care, going it alone, building a career first, or finding success late – there is no easy way to be an 'art monster' while also trying to raise a child.

In the absence of societal encouragement or approval, women have had to find their own ways through that tension, some of them not always admirable. Some, like Lessing, lost access to their children. The common narrative continues to be that she fully abandoned them without looking back – which says it all, really. Others had strained or distant relationships with their offspring. But many flourished, too, as did their children.

What these women all needed, Phillips concludes, was time. How they achieved that differed – Toni Morrison got up to write before her children woke, Le Guin didn't, because hers would always stir when she did. But, heroically, each of them endeavoured to find ways around it. Barbara Hepworth claimed that taking as little as half an hour a day for herself, 'to allow the images to build in one's mind', was enough to maintain her artistic consciousness while caring for triplets.

They also needed a sense of self. It is so easy to be entirely sublimated by motherhood, to allow your self to be annihilated. To demand boundaries, to assert that you have a right to make art: that requires strength and conviction. It is, as Phillips has it, a hero's journey.

To put the baby on the fire escape is not to literally leave your child out in the cold. But it is the ability to put the baby out of your mind for the time required to create something else. That's not to say you're immune to guilt. It can feel like a constant tug of push and pull, the need to be present for your child versus the desperate need to create. It is far from easy.

Many women know this – it is the tension at the heart of Sheila Heti's book *Motherhood*, in which her narrator eventually decides not to sacrifice her artist self through motherhood. There was a time when I feared every baby might be a book I didn't write. The proverbial 'pram in the hall' as the 'enemy of all good art' still haunts so many of us, though it is a nonsense. Furthermore, as Vinko and a long line of female artists before her have shown, the experience of motherhood also lends itself to groundbreaking works interrogating and interpreting it.

I left my baby to write this, when all he wanted was to nestle close to me and feed and sleep. While writing, my body has literally ached for him. This will ease with weaning, but that knowledge sits with the fact that I will only have so many of these days, and that I have never, not since he was born, been fully present for him, because there is a treacherous part of me that will always need to write. I believe that I have the sense of self to do it, but sometimes it can feel exhausting. The temptation to put down one's pen, or one's paintbrush, can be immense, but, as the Swedish artist and writer Emma Ahlqvist writes in her book *My Body Created a Human*, 'I don't want my child to grow up having the pressure of having a parent who has given up everything in their life for them.' She concludes that, 'Having limited time has made me realise what I really need in my life, and that is to make art.'

Of course, in order to keep going as a mother and an artist, you need an art world, or a publishing world, that is hospitable to both mothers and works about motherhood. Hettie Judah's *How Not to Exclude Artist Mothers (and Other Parents)* is a manifesto for change at every level, from art schools to studios to institutions and beyond. As she writes, 'When an artist discovers she is pregnant she should not immediately be gripped by the anxious prospect of having commissions cancelled, abandoning her studio practice and losing sight of a fruitful career. Parenthood should be the start, not the end of things.'

Feeling guilty for putting your baby in nursery? That suits the government just fine

(Or: In which we find some childcare, and I wonder who has the separation anxiety: me, or my son?)

In the end, it was Mariah who did it. I had been trying so hard not to cry, and in fact was feeling quite cheerful about the baby starting nursery and me reclaiming some precious time, which I am mostly planning to use by lying on the floor. Besides, the bairn is a socialite, so is thrilled to be hanging out with so many other babies. The first day of settling in went well. I was feeling buoyed. 'Until Always Be My Baby' came on, that is.

I wept. People said I would, but the force of the emotion surprised me. 'It can be hard for the mums,' the kindly staff had said. You're telling me. I thought I had got used to the mixed emotions that come with parenthood. I hadn't foreseen bawling at 90s pop hits. But I know that some songs will always be different for me now. They'll come on in shops when I am fifty or sixty or seventy and hit me with the full force of how it feels to love him and miss him at all the ages he has ever been.

A week earlier I had gone to Foyles to sign some books, and while I was waiting I asked a staff member in the children's section for a book on separation anxiety. The book she brought me was *Owl Babies*, a classic of decades' standing. In it, the baby owls wake up to find their mother gone. They suspect she is hunting for food for them, but still, they are scared ('I want my mummy!' is the constant refrain). Of course, she comes back. I almost started crying right there in the bookshop.

The question is, who has the separation anxiety: me or the baby? I said goodbye (you must always say goodbye, they say, rather than slipping out), waited in reception until the allotted twenty minutes were up, and returned to discover that he had been fine. This was a fact that I found both cheering and faintly disappointing. When he had a meltdown the next day, I felt that same mix in reverse: cheered that he does in fact need me, disappointed that I didn't get to go and have a coffee on my own.

'Mummy's back, Mummy always comes back,' I say to him. I think he knows it, because he has, after that one big cry, settled remarkably quickly. They do it very slowly at his nursery, so for the first four days I didn't make it past reception. Now, when I drop him off, he barely looks at me. He has a day of playing ahead of him.

Some people can be judgmental about childcare, even now, when both parents almost always need to work outside the home to support their children. There seems to be this persistent idea that it's always best for every child to be at home with their mother. The educational and social benefits of childcare are rarely highlighted. On the baby's first day, a staff member dressed as a dragon and danced for the babies to celebrate the lunar new year. I am simply never going to do that. Aside from it possibly being culturally insensitive, I am too tired.

I suspect the notion that nursery is something families pay for when they have no choice comes from the fact that the British state still heavily relies on the unpaid labour of mothers to keep the show running: this is so deeply ingrained that paid childcare is barely ever thought of as a right, more a slightly uncomfortable necessity. In other countries, people feel entitled to it in a way many don't here, because lots of us feel too guilt-tripped. It's a form of ambient gaslighting, really, and it works. Women cobble together the patchy hours (often with part-time work or help from relatives), and their careers pay a price. They are giving so much, yet there's a niggling notion that it still falls short. It can feel like playing a doomed game of Tetris, in which the different components of your life don't fit together properly, so there's always a little gap you feel guilty about.

(Despite suggestions the government might increase its childcare offer in England, I have little faith that anything it implements will be radical enough to drastically improve affordability and availability.)

In my case, the guilt thankfully didn't last. But I am lucky: he will go for two and a half days a week, and besides, I have been too ill to feel overly upset – we all caught a hideous cold the minute he enrolled, naturally. Still, it feels like a sea change. Suddenly, I have some time. It is a shock that I had not expected. As Rachel Cusk wrote: 'I realise that I had accepted each stage of her dependence on me as a new and permanent reality, as if I were living in a house whose rooms were being painted and forgot that I ever had the luxury of their use. First one room and then another is given back to me.'

Once I have stopped sneezing, I tell myself that I will embrace the new spaces in my life. I will work, mostly, but I will also catch up on reading, I will see friends, I will swim. (I tell myself this, but if my first day of freedom is anything to go by, I will spend it doing things for him: babyproofing our home, and buying him little jumpers from charity shops.)

At the same time, I feel a tug of sadness that the days where the only space we needed was the size of a bed, lit by a lamp that shone through the endless night, with him at my breast; my body the border to his world and his to mine. And I will cry all over again.

As parents, can we all agree that a bit of screen time for children is actually a good thing?

(Or: On the complete and utter joy of CBeebies)

As the baby turns one, I've been looking back at the past year – which seems somehow to have been both the longest and shortest of my life – and reflecting on what I've learned. I embarked upon parenthood thinking I was at least a little bit prepared in terms of what it involved, only for it to be made swiftly apparent that I am utterly clueless. In fact, one of the sharpest, most humbling lessons so far has been the dawning understanding that no one actually really knows what they are doing most of the time.

I suspect that before a baby arrives we all have some ideas about the sort of parents we are going to be, only to guiltily dispense with those 'principles' one by one as the child grows. This has never been more apparent to me than when thinking about screen time. How I laugh now at the sweet summer child who obnoxiously recommended the CBeebies Prom to my fellow NCT mums, keen to stress that of course I turned his bouncer to face away from the screen. I'm surprised the poor baby didn't get a crick in his neck from craning to see what was going on.

I gave up trying in the end. By the time he was six months old he had watched a fair bit of football and most of Wimbledon with my husband, and quite a lot of *Strictly* with my mother (neither of whom are as neurotic as me).

Guidance on screen time varies. American paediatricians – those voices of authority who loom over anything you Google about babies ever: 'Consult them! Consult them!' you are implored – say no screen time until eighteen months(!). In the UK, we are more realistic. The NHS and NICE recommend an upper limit of two hours a day. The Royal College of Paediatrics and Child Health (RCPCH) criticised the US guidelines, and the NCT stresses the benefits to parents and children, in that it helps give children downtime and their carers get things done around the house, which is code for 'drink a glass of wine on the sofa'.

Though I have written before about the pressure on mothers especially to entertain and educate their babies constantly, making everything a learning opportunity, at least in this one respect our health bodies and charities seem to recognise a more balanced approach is needed.

Of course, that doesn't mean we don't feel guilty. I have yet to hear a parent discuss screen time without it being in a hushed tone of someone admitting to a shameful secret. The baby has been through another period of illness, as well as adjustment to nursery, and TV has enabled him to rest and recuperate when he hasn't felt like playing. When a few months ago he was hospitalised, Disney songs kept him calm and still while the tubes and wires could do their work making him better. When he said 'bear', clear as a bell while watching a song from *The Jungle Book*, I thought, well, telly can't be all bad.

And yet the guilt persists. My husband, who is from a large family and whose first words were 'Joe Montana', argues that some of this is 'precious firstborn' syndrome. If you have more than one child, good luck trying to stop them from watching TV. He points out that he watched back-to-back *Ninja Turtles*, not to mention the four hours preceding *Ninja Turtles* while they waited for it to come on. 'I'm not talking about *Ninja Turtles*, though!' I wailed. 'I'm talking about the BBC Philharmonic Orchestra!'

Clearly, I need to get over myself. Which is why I think transparency about screen time is important, even if it means being judged. People treat it as though you're using it as a stand-in for a lovely countryside walk or a day at the museum, as opposed to 'quiet time'. A friend whose toddler has additional needs says that screen time is crucial for him to decompress after nursery.

My own brother is autistic, and coming across *Something Special* on CBeebies, which uses Makaton to help children with communication difficulties, actually made me feel quite tearful, as nothing like this existed when he was young. Yes, it's easy to see how too much screen time could affect development, but an all-or-nothing approach helps no one, especially not when you are desperately trying to make a seemingly simple supper of pasta and tomato sauce – which these days feels as ambitious as the coq au vin I used to do from scratch, pre-baby – without the bairn wreaking havoc.

So I acknowledge, with a full heart, that I have used TV to help me parent, and I feel incredibly grateful to the BBC. I now understand, as no doubt many, many of you did before me, why she is an 'Auntie' to so many of us. The quality of the programming for young children is astonishing, and all without having to expose them to advertising, which I loathe and which is my parental red line. Yes, having the theme tune to *Small Potatoes* (described as 'an animated series about a group of potatoes who sing songs in different genres') going round my head at 4 a.m. is not ideal, but I'll take it for the joy it gives my boy.

You have probably noticed that I've focused mostly on television, and that's because the other kind of screen time feels less benevolent. Come back to me when my toddler is bidding for *Postman Pat* memorabilia on eBay using my PayPal and has become prey to the YouTube algorithm, and perhaps we'll have a different sort of conversation. But for now the screen time in our lives all feels very gentle, wholesome and educational, and I feel ever so slightly less exhausted and overwrought.

What worked

- The Toy Project – a charity that recycles unwanted toys and sends them to children who need them, whether in refuges, hospitals, children's homes or abroad. The range available to customers is brilliant, too, and if you're in the London area it's well worth the trip. I get most of my stocking fillers there every Christmas.

- *Postman Pat: Special Delivery Service*. I will never forget the look on my son's face the first time he saw it, and despite the fact that Pat is pretty useless at his job, he remains a firm favourite.

- Melty Puffs. I finally got to a place where I was comfortable with him handling and eating bigger bits of food, and all thanks to the melty puff. Before I became a parent, I had assumed everyone was giving their baby cheesy Wotsits. These are an apparently healthier alternative, designed for young kids. I know a couple of mums who overdid it on the wine and ended up snaffling several packs of said puffs, but they are, in my opinion, bland as hell. They're fine for babies, but I think I'll stick to my favourite brand of fluorescent crisp.

- The baby's door bouncer was really coming into its own at this stage, as he was desperate to be on the move but wasn't crawling (we tend to be bum shufflers in my family). I have fond memories of the little Irish jig he used to do in it.

- The books *Peck Peck Peck* by Lucy Cousins, *I Want My Hat Back* by Jon Klassen and *Little Owl's Bedtime* by Karl

Newson. But most of all, Emma Dodd's *Me*. The way my son used to smile at and kiss the baby penguin melted my heart, and I've never met a baby that didn't love it.

What didn't

- This was a time of intense sleep deprivation, and the only way I survived was to go into another room with an eye mask and earplugs for a totally sensorily deprived snooze, while Tim watched the baby. Unfortunately, the cat worked out how to open doors, and decided that mornings were prime time for playing on my head.

- Sleep, food, bottles – you name it. Part of what was causing the sleep deprivation was that, after being so unwell, not to mention teething and separation anxiety, the baby had by this point reverted to wanting to breastfeed constantly, and was waking almost every hour throughout the night to do so. When I wasn't fantasising about checking into a hotel to catch up on some much-needed sleep, I was wondering how on earth I was going to get to a point when I could stop breastfeeding and gain some independence – not only for me, but also for him.

- The dramatic side effects of infant antibiotics, the details of which I won't go into in case you're eating breakfast.

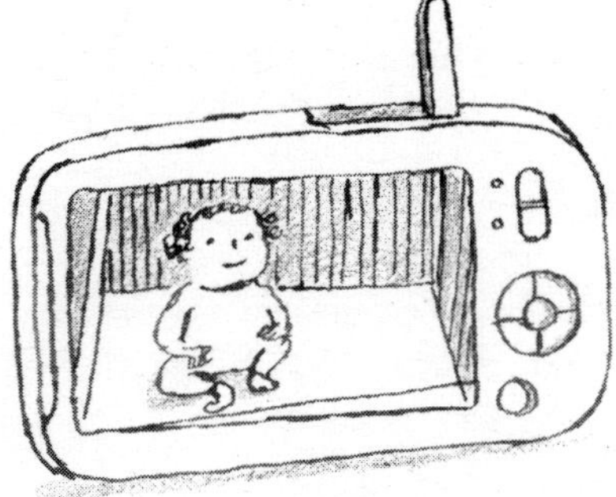

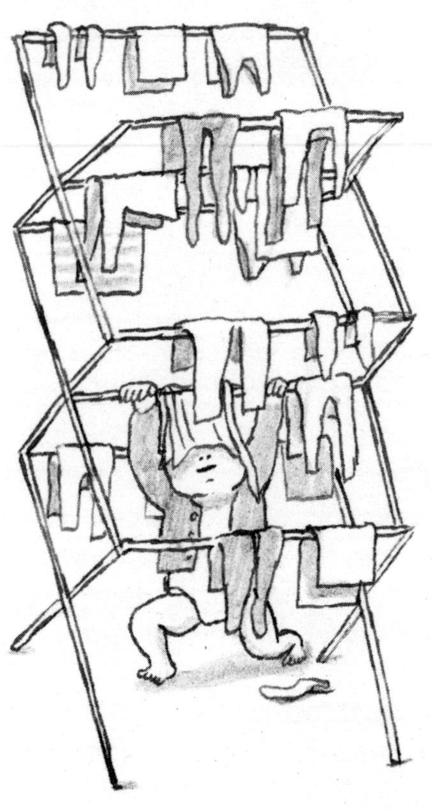

12–18 months

Stopping breastfeeding my baby offers a bittersweet relief

(Or: Reflecting on how my journey through mixed feeding was painful but beautiful)

It's more than a year since I had my baby and I'm still breastfeeding. If you read my first, furious column about it, you might be surprised: nursing was a challenge. We both cried for weeks. Sometimes I screamed in pain. The guilt I felt for using formula – despite my hungry pre-term baby's need for it – was matched only by the fury I felt at the professionals who treat exclusive breastfeeding as worth the sacrifice of a mother's mental health.

My mind boggles at some of the advice I was given: how I was instructed to pump after every feed, but no one thought to tell me that I needn't continue this indefinitely, compounding my distress and exhaustion; the lactation-promoting drug – which I did not take because one of the side-effects was depression – I was prescribed despite my milk coming in as normal on day three; the NCT breastfeeding 'expert' who said that the pain was because we were doing it wrong; my tiny baby who had not been in the womb long enough to fully develop his feeding reflex, with his tied tongue and his minuscule mouth opening and closing like a baby bird's as he struggled to latch, and I, his mother, bruised and bleeding. I finally had to steel myself to firmly tell the health visitor that exclusive breastfeeding was no longer realistic or desirable for either of us.

The benefits of breastfeeding are often overstated. A new University of Glasgow study may have made those who couldn't breastfeed feel even worse. The study has found that compared to formula-only feeding, breast- and mixed-fed babies are at a lower risk of having special educational needs. 'Yet,' says Dr Danya Glaser, visiting professor at UCL, and honorary consultant child and adolescent psychiatrist at Great Ormond Street children's hospital, 'correlation does not equal causation. The study has not been adequately controlled for the role of low socioeconomic status in both breastfeeding and SEN prevalence.' (It also struck me that babies who are premature or have undergone difficult births are at greater risk of learning disabilities. Establishing breastfeeding can also be more challenging with such babies.)

Research is to be welcomed, of course. As Joanna Wolfarth points out in *Milk: An Intimate History of Breastfeeding*, we have more scientific research on tomatoes than we do on breast milk. Many studies should be taken with a pinch of salt, nevertheless. And I would like to say, clearly and definitively to any new mother, read the chapter on breastfeeding in Eliane Glaser's *Motherhood: Feminism's Unfinished Business*, and liberate yourselves from guilt.

Another thing that can go to hell alongside guilt is the myth of nipple confusion. Mixed feeding is the reason that I am still breastfeeding. No one talks about it because new mothers are so infantilised that we are considered better off not hearing about it, in case we get any ideas. I'm sure I'd have given up sooner had my husband not shared the work of infant feeding, forming a wonderful bond with the baby in the process. Mixed feeding has enabled me to work, socialise, go to galleries and, most importantly, sleep. It has helped me live a full life while breastfeeding. It has been, for my family, the best of both worlds.

There have been moments this past year when the baby's need for my milk has felt annihilating, when my blood-sugar level has dipped so low I have almost lost consciousness. I have felt at times, to quote Elena Ferrante, 'like a lump of food … a cud made of a living material that continually amalgamated and softened its living substance to allow two greedy bloodsuckers to nourish themselves'.

At others, breastfeeding has felt miraculous, and I have come to understand that old religious fervour for it, felt flickers of divinity and of reverence. In periods of illness, he has taken the breast where he would take no other sustenance, and I have felt pride and relief in his return to health, and in our bond. I can see why people get romantic and emotional, why Wolfarth cried in front of Louise Bourgeois' sculpture *The Good Mother* – I stood in the same spot weeks after giving birth and cried too. Like her, it made me think of the bonds that nursing can create with the wider community. I will always feel a warm glow when I think of Karen, from Islington Breastfeeding Support, of my cousin Emily, who gave me 24/7 text advice while tandem feeding her children, and of Sue, the lactation consultant who changed everything.

Thirteen months on, and this morning, as I held my son to my breast, I felt a wave of love and loss. I am in the process of cutting down the feeds – slowly, to avoid too much of a hormone drop – and it's by no means emotionally straightforward. 'No one tells you how to stop,' my sister-in-law said, wryly, as she tried to wean her three-year-old. I do not want to breastfeed for that long – the baby has started nursery and besides, I'm going to Glastonbury without him – but there will be a mourning process.

Everywhere I look I seem to see mothers nursing their newborns, and I try not to stare, but I feel something akin to a craving, to be feeding a baby that small again, to be, in those short – or interminable – moments, his world. In *Milk*, Wolfarth writes of the Tintoretto painting *The Origin of the Milky Way*, based on a Roman retelling of the Greek myth of Hera, whose milk splatters across the sky and creates the stars (the cosmic dust of which is contained within all of us, an apt metaphor). The idea moves me. It makes me want to pay tribute to my own milk and the body that made it. Although it is time my son and I both looked outwards, for our universes to expand, I feel wistful. Despite its challenges, nursing him has been a privilege and a gift.

I once argued fiercely for child-free spaces. As a mother, I still believe in their sanctity

(Or: On how the pub became our second living room, but sometimes I just want to be around adults)

This morning I did something that I rarely do, for fear of inducing a full-body cringe the likes of which I have not experienced since, aged ten, I jumped on my dad's back in the local swimming pool only to discover that it wasn't him: I read one of my old columns. Written nearly a decade ago under the headline 'I'll drink to child-free pubs and cafes', my twentysomething self grumbles about the presence of kids in adult spaces.

Fast forward and I have a one-year-old who regards my local pub as an extension of his living room. I have sung him to sleep in the beer garden and breastfed him, rosé in hand, while sharing birth stories. Sometimes, I have looked up and seen an exclusion zone of empty tables around where we are sitting. Time makes hypocrites of us all.

There has been a lot of discussion about child-free spaces recently, with two reported plane incidents going viral. The first involved a pregnant woman being asked by cabin crew to clear up her children's popcorn crumbs, and the second, a grown man's tantrum about the presence of a crying baby on his flight, during which, after his fellow passengers told him he was shouting, he replied with the immortal: 'So is the baby! Did that motherfucker pay extra to yell?'

Both provoked fierce debate online that can be boiled down to, on the one hand, 'Crying babies are annoying and should not be in public. Being unable to soothe them is poor parenting', vs 'Children and babies are a part of society and they also cry. No one wants them to stop crying more than their own parents.' Although these factions could broadly be categorised along the lines of 'child-free/childless' people and 'childed' people (a word I dislike, but one that is becoming increasingly popular), many of us could see both sides.

I couldn't not laugh at the man's furious logic, because I have felt that, before and after becoming a parent. But motherhood has elevated my (already high) threat responses to the point where a large, angry man shouting at me and my baby in a confined space would almost certainly make me burst into tears, not to mention frighten the poor child. To intimidate babies and their mothers like that is unpleasant, to say the least.

Online, parents and child-free people often seem to be at war. Offline, however, in my personal relationships things feel a lot more cordial, perhaps because we love the people in our lives regardless of their reproductive status, or perhaps because all the beef is simply simmering, unarticulated, under the surface.

Since I became a parent, I've been having discussions with friends and readers about what it means to live a child-free life. They have made me think more deeply and empathically about how it feels to be part of a society where parenthood is the default journey when one does not have children. My colleague Helen Pidd's recent article about the child-free movement and its radical, pioneering spirit, as well as our series 'Why I don't have a child', added further to my understanding. The decision to be childfree is not always painless and can feel lonely. I can understand not always wanting to be reminded of that tough choice, or having the desire to feel like you're enjoying life unencumbered. Parents benefit from child-free spaces, too. I love to read a book alone in a pub or cafe, and my heart will sometimes sink at the sight of a crying baby when I have left my own at home for some vital alone time.

I don't take offence when people articulate a need for child-free spaces. When a child-free thirty-seven-year-old woman tells me that she doesn't really want to be around children all the time, I get it. 'But if you say that you have committed two massive, unforgivable crimes: not wanting kids (what is wrong with you?) and then not wanting to at least be involved with kids (you are a freak and must be a psychopath!),' she says.

I tell her that I always try to ask my child-free friends whether I should bring the baby along or not. 'Hanging out with kids introduces all the elements I struggle with: chaos, noise, endless tasks… Sometimes that's OK and it's fun, but I appreciate it when friends don't assume I'll want to do that,' she says, noting that you can never have a proper conversation with another adult when their child is around. It brings to mind the phone call with married-with-toddlers Magda in *Bridget Jones's Diary*: 'Bridget, hi! I was just ringing to say in the potty! In the potty! Do it in the potty!'

Though the UK could be more child-friendly, I do still believe in the sanctity of adult-only spaces that I argued for in my past column, and, to quote restaurant critic Marina O'Loughlin: 'Children shouldn't rule the roost anywhere, frankly, but restaurants least of all. I've endured too many longed-for, carefully planned moments totally bollocksed by them.'

I suppose it boils down to a need for kindness and empathy on both sides. We all started life as babies screaming from colic or explosive diarrhoea. Babies cry as a way of communicating, and being a part of humanity means that we can't always choose which other humans communicate with or around us. But when there's an exit that isn't 30,000 feet up in the sky, parents can also choose to take their baby through it.

To my friend who worries about becoming a parent: here are some things to hold on to

(Or: For Alex, who now has a beautiful baby girl)

I decided to write this column in the format of a letter. I wanted to set myself the writing challenge of citing some of the many positive things about having a baby without being saccharine, resorting to cliché or generalising, and the only way I could find was this way. It's addressed to one person, but I hope that those who find themselves at a similar crossroads take succour from it.

To my friend A,

When you sidled up to me at a party recently and confessed that you wanted to have a baby, we were both drunk. So when you said that you needed reassurance that it wouldn't be awful, because all you ever seem to hear about parenthood is negative, I probably didn't give you what you needed that night. I've been mulling over what you said ever since.

I read somewhere not long ago that children ruin your life. I do not feel this (I was at a party, for a start). You create a new life in that child, and with that baby, you get a new life, too. I look back on my old self with fondness, and a little indulgence. She had a lot of fun, but it was time for a new adventure. A baby is more than just an adventure, though: you're embarking on an epic quest that will hopefully see them safely into adulthood. We hear a lot about the obstacles we meet on the way and less about the wonders we encounter, so I wanted to say that: you will experience wonder the likes of which you can't imagine now.

The wonder seems mundane to other people, of course, and that's part of the problem. For example: my baby is doing this thing at the moment where he has started kissing his favourite characters in the books we read. Every time he does it I feel a soaring happiness that feels almost criminal, like I'm getting away with something. What I'm saying is that you can spend your whole life trying to be happy, taking up wild swimming or yoga or microdosing LSD or having therapy, but, for me, nothing has come close to the feeling of watching my child launch himself at a drawing of a fluorescent pink simian who has just learned the importance of saying sorry to an elephant with hurt feelings.

It's not just your happiness, either: it's theirs. Giving your baby a lovely day feels genuinely fulfilling for you, but less selfishly, joy has been created for them, and the amount of happiness on this planet has increased. It may be by a tiny amount, in a global context, but to that child, it is everything.

Another one of those clichés is that it's 'a love unlike any other' – a nonsense, because no love is like any other. What I will say is that it's a love that feels primal and molecular. It has a before, and an after. Before I felt this love, I could imagine it, because like most humans I am capable of empathy, but I had not lived with it. The life I had before I got to feel this love feels like less of a life. That is not to say that I believe people who are not parents live less meaningful lives. I don't, at all. But my life has greater meaning to me, for loving him.

And of course, his life has meaning. He exists! It still feels wild and miraculous that this should be the case, and not just because it wasn't the easiest birth.

(Try not to worry about the birth. We usually hear the horror stories, and they are important, but good births happen, too.) Becoming a mother – and giving birth – has enhanced my feelings of solidarity with other women. It is a solidarity that is physical, intellectual, emotional and political. It is also historical. I feel empathy with women who lived and died many centuries before I even existed. And that has expanded my heart and my mind.

When I became a mother, it was as though all the mothers in my life, even peripherally, received some sort of alert signal, and rallied. Even the mothers of friends of mine, whom I rarely see, sent gifts and messages. Other mothers brought meals or gave breastfeeding support or medical advice. Their well wishes, guidance and care held me in an embrace that lasted for many months after the birth. My own mother's embrace, and my father's, not to mention my extended family's, have kept me going.

We are used to hearing about how motherhood limits and constricts your life, less so about how it can expand it. A world of other mothers – other parents, actually – has revealed itself to me. I have always believed that life is fundamentally about human relationships, and having a baby has enhanced mine. I love my husband more than ever.

Parenting has also allowed me to experience childhood again. I always wanted to give someone else a childhood. My wide-eyed little boy is at the stage where he is simply in love with the world, and that love is thrillingly unconditional (he is beside himself every time he sees a pigeon). It is a privilege to witness, and it makes me determined to maintain it for him as much as I am able, because his laugh is the best sound that I have ever heard.

A note about sleep: you will be OK – you've had enough wild nights to know you can cope. And you can get your body back, whatever that might mean to you. I feel I have (ish). As for your career, it's normal to worry. I speak only for myself when I say that I wish I had spent less time fretting beforehand about how I would write. I have far less time, now, but I'm still writing. Even a paragraph a day adds up to a novel, eventually.

There is so much untapped joy, hilarity and love there waiting for you, and I hope I've given you a small glimpse of some of it to hold on to.

Can we call time on the 'doesband' doing 'daddy daycare'? Fathers are way past that

(Or: On how many millennial men are parenting differently)

Are you a 'doesband'? The latest irritating portmanteau refers to a husband who parents his own children. 'A doesband has his own hectic job, but still does his fair share at home Without Being Asked,' writes Harriet Walker, the *Times* journalist who coined the term. 'A doesband knows where the Calpol is and when ballet kit is needed … He gets up with the children and does bedtime; he feeds them, bathes them, does the school run; knows when their nails need to be cut and that behind their ears can get gunky.'

I hate the term, but Walker makes a salient point: that men who share childcare equally with their partners, including the mental load, are still rarer than they should be. There are more and more female breadwinners, but according to the Office for National Statistics, women still do 60 per cent more unpaid work than men. Walker writes about staying awkwardly silent during conversations with other women about their useless partners. It can feel like boasting to go into just how much your male partner does (I'm only discussing heterosexual relationships here).

Since having a baby, I've been depressed by how little some men seem to get away with doing when it comes to their own children, and how normalised that is. Take the loathsome phrase 'Daddy daycare', or the fact that my husband is frequently congratulated for taking his own son out for a walk – something that has literally never happened to me. I feel lucky to have a partner who took four months of shared parental and annual leave, who feeds (we combi-fed, which set the tone from the start), changes, comforts, plays, cooks, shops, sorts the childcare payments, night-weaned the baby and – the worst task of all – deals with the nappy bins. Yet I shouldn't feel lucky, it should be normal.

On the bright side, lots more men are what used to be called 'involved fathers', while also trying to hold down full-time work. Seeing how challenging that can be has made me reflect how, in our capitalist system, men can't have it all either. For many, being able to work from home during the pandemic has been a game changer. 'I don't think women are inherently better caregivers than men,' says Alex Marsh, a thirty-nine-year-old market researcher with two daughters, aged nine and twelve. He tells me that he has always strived to do his share, remembering how the midwife 'wrote "hands-on dad" on her notes, as though that was remarkable' when he and his wife said they shared the nappy changing. Alex was the 'night duty' parent, but was still working in London all week.

Now that he only goes into the office twice a week, he is able to read his kids bedtime stories every night, cook most of their meals and handle their school admin: 'And I love it,' he says. Alex says he doesn't feel that exceptional among his peers, except maybe in terms of the cooking, but he worries that they are a minority. 'There are still a lot of relationships out there where the woman is expected to do more, simply because she is a woman.'

A friend who works in tech, a similarly hands-on dad, doesn't feel rare either. He finds the term 'doesband' infantilising. He's messaging me back at 3.05 a.m. while trying to settle his toddler daughter and says the majority of fathers he knows are equal parents. In his industry, it's considered commonplace: he got four months of paid paternity leave.

'I still notice a huge generational legacy in behaviour,' he says. His grandparents and parents have been surprised by how dedicated he and his partner are to parenting equally.

That's not to say it's easy: 'There's no getting around that it's draining and runs you into the ground,' he says. 'In the early stages there's anger and frustration.'

My friend's talk of the early stages makes me think that perhaps some couples succeed at equal parenting right off the bat, while others negotiate and learn as they go. Steph Douglas, who runs the thoughtful gift company Don't Buy Her Flowers and has three children, says: 'It's been a "journey" that has involved me trying to understand why I was so resentful and unhappy after we had kids.' She found the 'fair play' method – a system that helps couples share household chores equally – key in making their parenting genuinely more equal rather than simply giving her husband a list of tasks. As well as now sharing much of the parenting, her partner is in the school WhatsApp group – they succeeded in signing up all the dads after she noticed it was only mothers.

Some of us might move in circles where equal parenting is the norm, but the stats tell a different story. There is cause for hope, though. While hands-on dads have always existed, they are becoming more commonplace among younger generations of parents, and policy – especially in terms of paternity leave – needs to catch up. Women seem less inclined to put up with an unfair division of labour and a heavy mental load, which is sexist and in many cases no longer makes financial sense. I enjoy the TV comedy *Motherland*, and have seen that, sadly, the useless, absent husband in it reflects the reality in some households. But millennial fathers I speak to repeatedly highlight how retrograde and depressing the wimpy stay-at-home dad character Kevin is. He simply does not resonate with younger parents, and though there is still a long way to go, that can only be a cause for hope. As for the term 'doesband', it can get in the bin with the nappies.

British parents need to adapt to climate chaos – but not by abandoning the great outdoors

(Or: On the importance of weather)

Like all children, I hated rainy days. What I didn't realise until I had my own baby was how my parents probably hated them, too. Cooped up, whingeing babies can make cooped up, whingeing babies of their adult caregivers, too. 'Get outside every day,' people tell you, but you find yourself and the child all wrapped up and ready to go and standing in a doorway watching the showers come down in biblical sheets. A 2016 study that found that British children spend less time outdoors than prison inmates started to make a little bit more sense.

I have sung a lot of 'Singin' in the Rain' this past winter, and then spring, but sometimes I've been crying on the inside. I don't get seasonal affective disorder, but by April my spirits were starting to feel low. The weather feels personal now, in a way that it never did before, when I could hunker down with a book or a film or a glass of red wine and a record. Now stormy weather means trying to find endless entertainment for a baby who loves nothing more than being outside and watching the wind shake the leaves. It couldn't have been more different than the spring we brought him into the world: our postpartum euphoria as we walked him through sunlit streets, long lunches of seafood pasta while he slept in the pram, pink blossom falling like snowflakes on the day we registered his birth. This year, it's been so wet that he's only just touched grass.

It got me thinking about how weather and climate radically alter our experience of parenting and the culture of parenthood, depending on where on the planet we find ourselves. Before we had the baby, we used to go to Greece, and in my twenties I spent a year living in Italy. In both cases, I was always struck by the Mediterranean attitude to parenting, the children out playing far past British bedtime, as their parents dined and socialised nearby. I always felt that I wanted to be like that – not least because a later bedtime surely means a more civilised wake-up time – but, as well as the weather, it's a challenge in a country that does not treat public space in the same way. The piazza shapes parenting, as it shapes many aspects of Italian life.

The Arctic survival parenting of Sami reindeer herders is another example of how climate shapes family life. Children are taught independence from a young age as a way of building resilience in a hostile climate – children choose when they eat and when they sleep, curling up for a nap wherever they feel like it. 'Me and the children can nap on an all-terrain vehicle, snowmobile, under a rain cover in a trailer or in our van', a woman who married into a Sami family told the BBC. Families don't follow a schedule; the terms are set by the natural environment.

Now that things have brightened up, I have vowed to work towards helping my boy to learn to nap outside on a rug. Yesterday, in the playground, I met a Portuguese nanny who had put her charge face down on a blanket on the large circular nest swing and covered her with a coat. When I asked the woman how she had managed to get her to sleep so soundly, her response indicated that a child refusing to nap was not really an option. They sleep better outside, she said.

Scandinavians are inclined to agree. They're famous for leaving sleeping babies in prams in the street, and will bundle them up and allow them to nap outside even in sub-zero temperatures. Nursery schools will put the children down in the garden, the theory being that the children are less likely to catch viruses than if you have them all sharing the same room.

One piece of Finnish research found that babies slept longer outdoors than indoors.

Perhaps my countryside roots are manifesting in my resistance to being an urban, ‘indoor’ parent, or perhaps being outside just feels more natural to me. In an evolutionary sense, we are supposed to be outdoors, and, just as how babies relax during movement speaks to our nomadic past, there must be an atavistic desire to spend time in the open air.

In the climate emergency, however, outdoor parenting is going to become more challenging than ever as weather becomes more extreme. The heatwave last summer, when I took the baby out only in the early mornings and late evenings, though it hit 28°C by 7 a.m., gave me a glimpse of things to come. Will the next few decades see London become unlivable for the very young and the very old? Our architecture is not built for heat as it is in warmer countries, and I’ll never forget the hellish week we spent breastfeeding under a fan, stuck together by a film of sweat. Periodically I would sponge down both the baby and Mackerel, our poor, panting cat, with flannels cooled in the fridge. We even considered putting him on Mackerel’s special pet cooling mat.

Society will need to adapt, or British children will end up more cooped up than ever. I am immensely privileged to live in a place where the local government has prioritised shaded playgrounds, paddling pools and sprinkler areas, so that all children, regardless of whether they have access to a garden, can enjoy the summer. I can’t wait to introduce him to the joy of water play, but perhaps it’s time to think about a life that looks beyond the paddling pool to a closer engagement with nature. In the meantime, let’s just hope the weather holds up.

My irrational hatred of one *Postman Pat* character is a tribute to the genius of British children's TV

(Or: In which I have spent far too much time watching CBeebies)

There's a character on *Postman Pat* that I hate, passionately. Bill Thompson, the child of Alf and Dorothy, is a snarky little sod with an attitude problem. There's a part in an episode about a treasure hunt, where he says 'I'd be finished by now if I didn't have to wait for you slowcoaches', which invokes in me an almost physical loathing. Even the *Postman Pat* fandom page describes him as 'conceited'. I've spent so much time watching *Postman Pat* with my baby that I've conjured up *Succession*-worthy backstories to explain Bill's flawed personality – is it the pressure of being promised his dad Alf's farm from an early age?

This is what happens with children's television, once you become a parent and suddenly find yourself watching it. You know you're watching something created for children, but you cannot help but impose onto it an adult sensibility. For example, people often remark that *Postman Pat* is objectively a terrible postman – always losing the thing he is supposed to be delivering. I counter that since Royal Mail privatisation and the transformation of his role into 'special delivery', he is probably on a zero-hours contract, not to mention constantly being asked to do things, such as flying a helicopter or catching a pony, that are well beyond a usual postman's duties. My father, when visiting, pointed out that Pat being constantly tracked on an app by Ben in the office is an accurate portrayal of the kind of surveillance capitalism many workers are now forced to contend with.

We may enjoy picking holes in what our children watch, but parents in Britain are immensely privileged to have such high-quality children's television, especially the BBC, whose CBeebies channel and programmes are world leaders. It's one of the few things the UK can feel proud of on the global stage at the moment. That's not to say that other countries' offerings are poor – I grew up with *Sesame Street* (the US), and we love *Bluey* (Australia). TV adaptations of books such as *Barbapapa* (France) and the *Moomins* (Finland) are rightfully canonical. And of course work by people of many nationalities airs on CBeebies – one of our favourites, the hilarious animated series *Small Potatoes*, was created by American *Sesame Street* writer Josh Selig and also aired on Disney in the US.

So I'm open to the notion that I may be culturally biased in thinking that our programming is superlative. I'm not sure, however, that there are many nations in the world that have their finest stage actors delivering lines such as 'Hello Tombliboos!' with the same gravitas as 'Out, out, brief candle!' (Derek Jacobi), or juggling *Wolf Hall* with being the voice of an animated rabbit (Mark Rylance). And from a diversity perspective it feels radical: I have become quite emotional seeing how CBeebies includes children with disabilities.

British children's television is internationally exported, with programmes such as *Teletubbies* becoming an enduring international sensation, *In the Night Garden* relying heavily on global sales and even Quentin Tarantino saying he loves *Peppa Pig*. I suppose that's the thing about children's television – whoever you are, if you're a parent, you're probably watching it.

Which is one of the reasons why it's surprising it doesn't have a thriving critical climate: it's as worthy of scrutiny as any gallery opening or work of fiction, or indeed, adult TV. One of the few writers to turn their critical attention to it was Charlie Brooker, whose *Screenwipe* series was a characteristically intelligent and caustic examination, but that was fifteen years ago, and a one-off. Perhaps it's not considered serious enough to be worthy of consideration, or there's a residual misogyny about it, as something children 'watch with mother'. Yet it shapes the identities, values and interests of the next generation.

If anything, revelations about the darker side of children's television and the abusive crimes of some of its past stars show that the industry and its output should be subjected to a healthy amount of adult scrutiny as part of our wider cultural experience, rather than sequestered, dismissed or ignored. Perhaps there's an assumption that the readership isn't there for regular print reviews. Personally, I would gobble up a sarcastic essay on the hideous modern incarnation of *Peter Rabbit*, perhaps placing Beatrix Potter in a colonial context. A piece the *Guardian* ran on *Bluey* last year was, in my opinion, a tour de force.

Last year, the government pulled a £44 million fund designed to support the sector, and the BBC is facing budget cuts. The societal neglect of children's programming is partly behind why kids are deserting public service media in favour of YouTube and TikTok, and there is a real risk that distinctly British programmes for young viewers could vanish from screens and be replaced with imported shows.

More investment in the industry so that it can foster diverse creative talent, and the big ideas to compete with the streaming platforms, is crucial. But also, I think, our cultural attitude to children's content needs to change. At the moment, I don't think as a nation we truly appreciate the joy and innovation that goes into the work that is beamed into our homes every single day.

I may hate Bill Thompson, but I'll put up with him to see how that programme makes my little boy laugh with delight. As a family, we'd be lost without *Postman Pat*, and I suspect we're not alone.

The magic of holidays as a new parent? They're like time travel back to childhood summers

(Or: In which my boy sees the sea for the first time)

The people who design travel cots belong in prison. I'm generally in favour of restorative justice and rehabilitation, but for this I'll make an exception.

We are luckier than most, in that the baby will sleep on the hard bit of plywood that's supposed to pass for a mattress, but he does need a few pats on the bum to settle, and unless you are Stretch Armstrong (a contemporary reference there for you, kids) this is all but impossible. Likewise, lowering the baby (or in our case, large toddler) into the cot, which if you're a woman of average height involves squatting over one of the corners and hoping you don't bash your crotch on it so that your swearing wakes them up, something which definitely hasn't happened to me – ever. Basically, they are designed for babies who are heavy sleepers, and tall men.

If I sound grumpy, it's because we've just been on our first seaside holiday as parents, so travel cots are fresh in my mind. Though I opened with a negative, that first time your child sees the sea – if he or she is lucky enough to get there – is something very special. I knew he would love it, but I wasn't prepared for how much. I have written before about how parenthood allows you to experience childhood again and, as it turns out, this very British seaside holiday conjured for me many happy memories: of crabbing and paper sandcastle flags and fingers playing with the surface of rock pools, the soft, spongy feel of green seaweed beneath your toes, the roughness and smell of its black counterpart. It was like travelling in time, and has given me some of the happiest moments that I have ever known.

Holidays change when you are a parent. The packing and unpacking of bags feels almost constant. The volume of stuff that you have to bring is astonishing. The timing and smoothness of the journey becomes a lot more important, so when, for example, the air-conditioning is broken (as it was on both train journeys – thanks South Western!) it doesn't just feel uncomfortable but actually dangerous. As for flying, we haven't done that yet, but our NCT WhatsApp group has seen people sharing the minutiae of their journeys – what to do about bottles, which toys to pack to entertain their child, what to do if they have a massive nappy explosion. I'm grateful for this information from the parents braver than I – until quite recently, I couldn't face the prospect.

Mine is a well-travelled generation (five times more than our grandparents, according to one survey), and not having been abroad much growing up, I was lucky enough to be able to do so in my twenties. But our pre-term baby took a while to adjust to life outside the womb, and we've had a hard time with illness, so we cocooned ourselves for longer than many. There were times during my maternity leave that it felt almost as if we were 'wasting' it by staying at home.

A good friend went to ten countries during her maternity leave – including Argentina and Japan. She works hard and this was their opportunity to travel as a family. Of course, at times I felt jealous, especially over winter, as I pounded the pavements around my house for the thousandth time in the driving rain. But I also thought: all power to her for being so intrepid, though she feels guilty: 'I'm waiting for him to be an eco warrior when he grows up and hate us (you have to hate your parents for something).'

We are not the first generation to have travelled – a friend of mine was taken to Tibet as a baby – but I think we are the first generation to take it for granted. Not only that, but we risk our children turning to us and asking us, given the climate emergency, how we felt that we could justify ourselves. So in a way, not fancying a trip to Crete in August with a newborn (something a friend described as 'hell') has been good for our carbon footprint. It's a shame UK holidays are so expensive. Some London nurseries do day trips to the seaside, but every child deserves a holiday.

As well as being a matter of privilege and finances, I suspect travelling as a parent is down to temperament. I have learned that I am not one of those laid-back, gung-ho mothers. I will probably never take my child backpacking. Even the more remote Greek islands that I love are off limits for now. Yet the seaside trip has made a holiday abroad feel possible. I want a short flight, a nearby airport, a decent hospital and reasonable temperatures, but I'm starting to feel more optimistic.

That, I am coming to understand, is one of the lessons of parenthood. Things can seem hard, impossible even, and in the moment that feeling gives the impression of being permanent. It never is. When people say 'it gets easier', this is what they mean. Sometimes you try things and they don't work out, and these setbacks can shake your confidence. But often, like our little seaside trip, they do, and you can feel the world being returned to you, wider and more brimming with potential than before. Holidays may not be the same, but the joy of seeing the sea through your child's eyes makes up for the fact that you may have opted for a trip to Robin Hood's Bay as opposed to hiking in Peru. Perhaps the time will come that I feel brave enough. They'll have to design a better travel cot first, though.

I'll never be a true hippie parent, but I can learn a lot from summer festival-goers

(Or: On going to Glastonbury)

Every festival season, I think about something the writer Nell Frizzell once said to me during an interview about being the child of hippies and being taken to Womad, the international arts festival. She described it as 'standing in a field next to your dad wearing a bumbag, and thinking, "Oh, I've seen enough men from Kazakhstan playing fiddles."' It never fails to make me laugh, because not only have I lived that experience (though it was my mum who took me to Womad), but because it comically captures that feeling of your parents dragging you along to something that they insist you'll love when, really, you're there because they want to be.

I'm still recovering from Glastonbury – my first trip away from my son, and, it turns out, the perfect choice for that purpose, because there was so much going on that I couldn't focus on worrying about the distance between us. And it turns out that parenthood prepares you well for the chaos and squalor: could I handle very little sleep and quite a lot of exposure to human faeces? Absolutely. Am I inured to unpredictable behaviour, strange meals at odd hours and weird bursts of overwhelming emotion? Also, yes.

I was never going to take my son to Glastonbury, because I wanted that time for myself, but I didn't really have any thoughts about those who choose to take their children to large festivals until I saw first-hand what a miserable time some babies were having. On arrival I was almost immediately confronted by the sight of a near-naked newborn being carried through a campsite.

I try as much as possible not to judge other parents, but when, after midnight, you see a baby in ear defenders being hauled in a cart through a crowd of adults, all of whom are off their faces, while the infant cowers under a blanket, it doesn't really seem in their best interests. A couple of times I saw parenting that shocked me. 'It's really not OK,' one young woman said to me, near tears, about one especially distressed baby.

Still, I'm not saying these people were categorically bad parents. We've all misjudged situations, been overly optimistic and ended up regretting it. Perhaps these parents spent all day at the Kidzfield – which has amazing entertainment and where the National Childbirth Trust is on hand to help with feeding, bathing, and changing – and found they couldn't find their way back to their camper van. I noticed the kids having the worst time didn't seem to be the hippie kids. The hippie kids you see at Womad and Glastonbury largely seem to be having a blast.

The happiest baby I saw all weekend was in a tipi in the Healing Felds with her mum, having a lovely, peaceful time. I also loved seeing the older kids, who reminded me of the ones I grew up around. You know the type: beautifully and rambunctiously feral, with ratty, long hair bleached by the sun, bare feet, weather-beaten faces. You can tell they live off-grid in Cornwall or Wales, spend all their time outdoors and scarcely know what the internet is. If my experience is anything to go by, let's just say there's a chance that they're not all up to date with their immunisations, and that really isn't OK; and, as I wrote in an article in 2017 about the hippie revival, they definitely face significant embarrassment in school and social settings. But in terms of the values that they are raised with, they are caring and kind and progressive. Often, the world that isn't comes as quite a shock.

Festivals are important for kids, I think, because they show diverse groups of people coming together in a largely harmonious way to engage with music and culture. They teach children about costume and play, and allow them to explore the outdoors safely away from screens. Recognising that modern parents are especially keen to continue going to them, festivals have become more child-friendly than ever, with Womad having a whole World of Children and Camp Bestival being entirely conceived of as a family-friendly festival-cum-camping holiday, with a plethora of activities and even a CBeebies bedtime story tent.

And they're important for parents, too. Some people would have you believe that your life is over when you have children. Festivals prove that you can still do things, albeit a bit differently. Though I didn't have my child with me, and was very much 'partying as a verb', I was still such a mum: making sure unaccompanied children made it out of the toilets OK, forming a human barrier to protect a crying teenage girl from a drunken oaf, carrying around a mini first-aid kit and a little sandwich bag of sliced orange for my pre-mixed Negroni.

Seeing the hippie kids of Glastonbury also made me question my own parenting, something that is healthy to do from time to time. Do I want my child to live a largely urban, indoor life, or am I interested in giving him something closer to my own childhood? We know from the children of the counterculture that hippie parents don't always get it right – while researching my first novel, which is on this very topic, I read some harrowing accounts, and would particularly recommend the book *Wild Child: Girlhoods in the Counterculture* edited by Chelsea Cain; but nor am I convinced that modern urban environments are always the best, either.

And so, like thousands before me, I have come away simultaneously shattered and enlivened, feeling that I have much to think about. Perhaps I'll want to change our lives, or perhaps I'll come back to earth, go back to how things were, and forget that other ways of living are possible. Until the next one, of course.

Art is a natural impulse, and babies are born critics: no wonder they love Van Gogh

(Or: On choosing paintings for the baby's room)

I'll admit I felt quite vindicated when I read of a new study this week that found that babies like Van Gogh. It seems he's as popular with the under-ones as he is with adults, or, more accurately: the adult preference for his work is mirrored in babies, suggesting certain biases in what we choose to look at are already present in infancy and carry over into adulthood. When choosing art for the baby's room, I looked at work created for that purpose, and almost all of it was saccharine and of poor quality. So I decided on fine art instead. I thought for a long time about which images to choose, wanting something that reflected what I thought he would enjoy, rather than my own specific taste. In the end I opted for *The Starry Night*, feeling instinctively that he would appreciate its mesmeric swirls as he drifts off to sleep.

The other two I chose were the brightest Jackson Pollock that I could find, and a pleasingly exuberant landscape by David Hockney. (It hardly needs explaining that these are posters that I am talking about. Were they actual originals, I would be writing this from my villa in the Luberon.) Before you pull me up on the lack of representation of female artists, I keep meaning to move the Lee Krasner in the hall in there, and I felt Georgia O'Keeffe was too vaginal, though I suppose babies should sometimes be reminded of where they are from ('She always rejected that interpretation of her work,' I said to my husband, when he remarked upon the print in the bathroom. 'Be real,' he said, 'It's a vag.'). And so the only female artist represented is my mother, Anna, with her beautiful painting of the bay at Naoussa, Paros. It turns out that this was a good choice, too, as the study found that infants gaze longer at stretches of sky.

I can't imagine living my life without art, or remember a time when I haven't enjoyed looking at it or making it. Children are natural artists, lacking the self-consciousness of adults in their desire for self-expression. It is such a human impulse, to make a mark. It is why I find the phrase 'My five-year-old could have done that' so tedious, and the book *Why Your Five Year Old Could Not Have Done That: Modern Art Explained* by Susie Hodge so inspired in its title. Children may lack the critical thought and talent of well-trained adult artists, but their playfulness, sense of imagination and humour are qualities that the adult artist retains, and can make their work captivating. I occasionally see grown-ups mocking their children's pictures and their lack of figurative resemblance to their subjects in a way that comes across as superior and occasionally cruel. It's OK to have a giggle occasionally, of course, but if you respond negatively to your child's work enough times they will stop making it. Besides, how utterly passé to view an ability to create a true likeness of the world as the only measure of artistic quality.

Of course, you can go too far the other way. My mother kept bags and bags of my childhood finger paintings, which she then tried to pass on to me in my early twenties. Funnily enough I didn't feel as sentimental about this juvenilia as she did, and there ensued a brutal cull. I may joke, but actually I strongly suspect that her ceaseless support of my creative work has given me the inner confidence to lead the life of a writer in adulthood, not to mention validated that crucial impulse, crushed out of so many of us, to make tangible the ideas in your mind.

Just look at the Young Artists' Summer Show, either in person at the Royal Academy or via the virtual exhibition online. The imagination on display, the humour. Where else could you see a crisp sandwich, a cat made of clouds, a narwhal that can communicate with the dead, a boy's baby sister, an abstract interpretation of the Lake District and a portrait of Richard Ayoade? One of my favourite pictures, by Nico, aged seven, bears the legend: I DON'T WANT TO ENTER THE ROYAL ACADEMY ART COMPETITION and shows a magnificent use of colour and a small, very funny grumpy face. Nico's witty rejection of the mainstream art establishment shows great promise in terms of a future career.

What I love the most when I look at these paintings is how happy they make me feel. Art can be pain, of course – without the latter we could not have the former – but it can also be joy. Unfortunately we are in a political climate where the appreciation and creation of art is so often dismissed as pretentious or navel-gazing, and creative subjects are deemed useless. Which is why we so desperately need that joy, and should try to recapture as much of it as we can for ourselves.

There's a video of my boy, only a few weeks old, gazing in amazement at the black and white outlines of a Keith Haring picture printed onto a 'sensory strip' (made by the company Etta Loves especially for newborns). The way his face changed as he absorbed the shapes: it still amazes me now. Van Gogh, I believe, understood this, which is why in a letter to his younger brother he wrote about the godlike nature of the child's gaze: 'I think that I see something deeper, more infinite, more eternal than the ocean in the expression of the eyes of a little baby when it wakes in the morning and coos or laughs because it sees the sun shining on its cradle. If there is a "ray from on high", perhaps one can find it there.'

Having a baby does mess with your memory. I'm glad I recorded the truth – good and bad – in real time

(Or: On 'baby brain')

How old was your baby when he started sleeping through?' asked a friend recently. She is in the trenches with her newborn, who will only sleep on her – an affliction that has the potential to push parents to the brink of madness, and for which they have yet to find a cure. I recalled that it was eight weeks, if you count sleeping through as five hours or more, but I didn't have the heart to tell her. I only remember, I think, because I was well rested enough to make decent memories.

People, readers included, took great joy in telling me that it wouldn't last, and they were right: it didn't. Though because of it, I can scarcely remember the winter at all. The baby was constantly unwell and we had entered the sort of co-sleeping situation that saw neither of us get much rest. For his part, he was waking for milk every hour; and for my part, I couldn't get a sentence from *Your Baby Week By Week* out of my head. The line was something like: 'Imagine how bad you'd feel if your baby died because you co-slept with them.' I can't remember it word for word now, but at the time it beat its way through the membrane of my troubled slumber to form a haunting refrain that meant any rest I was getting was of even poorer quality and thus, conversely, meant I was probably more likely to have an accident during my waking hours. (I should add here that I have great respect for the book's author Professor Caroline Fertleman and her co-writer Simone Cave, and say that I met the former when she was briefly my son's consultant and was genuinely starstruck. Some people turn to putty when they meet pop stars; for others, it's paediatricians.)

Memory is a strange thing. People, often mothers themselves, use the phrase 'baby brain' to describe that maddening inability to know where your car is parked or what that word is, or what the thing was that you went upstairs for. There is evidence that birth and the postpartum experience can affect our memories (but as the book *Mother Brain* by Chelsea Conaboy points out, there is very little research into baby brain in new fathers). In rats, memory appears to improve around the time of weaning and actually it seems that motherhood is beneficial for their brains in the long term. In women, we know that the hippocampus shrinks during pregnancy and the postpartum period. We also know that sleep deprivation affects our ability to encode memories in the hippocampus, which is perhaps why this past winter is recalled only in a series of flickering impressions: the sound of the machine delivering oxygen to my son, crying in a charity shop after we were discharged (but no recollection of the song that made me cry), the sight of his face when he touched snow for the first time, the theme tune to *Strictly Come Dancing*, which my mother watched while he sat beside her in the bouncer. Most of it is just darkness.

Similarly with the postpartum period: I remember how my mother tenderly brushed the knots from my hair, which had become so matted from writhing during labour that it wasn't until she was able to get to me, three weeks after the baby was born, that it could be untangled. Not because my husband couldn't do it, but because it hadn't occurred to me to ask him. There are some things that only mothers do. And I remember thinking, perhaps with that writerly impulse: this is something. I will remember this. I can remember the blood, the sound of my little baby's 'moth breath', as Sylvia Plath has it, and his hormone-drunk father saying, exuberantly, one day after coming home from the hospital: 'Let's have another one!'

My mother says no one remembers birth or the days that come after it, because if they did they wouldn't have more children. It serves an evolutionary purpose, she believes. And I can see what she is getting at, when I think about the pain of my labour, a pain so bad I said I would jump out of the window. I haven't forgotten exactly, but its edges have been blunted.

Perhaps this is why older people, when they give parenting advice, can sound so glib, so blasé. They might remember some of the details, but they are dulled. The immediacy of the experience has faded with time. It's one of the reasons why I admire my dad, because when I ask him what he did about such and such a problem, or at what age and stage I hit such and such milestone, he simply confesses that he can't remember. Rather than be didactic about it despite his vague recollections, he is honest about the gaps in his memory. Those prone to unsolicited parenting advice despite long having retired from active duty would do well to follow his example.

Writing this column has been one of the best things that I've ever done, and the only thing for which I've ever been regularly recognised by strangers. This isn't a boast: I'm no celebrity. It is in all the places you would expect: the playground, the breastfeeding group. But the thing people always say to me is: 'You write it exactly how it is.' It is only after months of doing this that I have understood how little of early parenthood is written in real time, for understandable reasons. But to reconstruct it in retrospect is to always lose something in the recounting. I read my early column about breastfeeding now and I can barely recall the pain and torment I felt. Which is why it's important that I wrote it. To remember. And so that those parents less able or inclined to record everything in writing from three weeks postpartum (because they are not insane!) remember too.

What worked

- Night weaning. My husband took a week off work and heroically night-weaned the baby, and we went from him waking every hour to some nine-hour stretches. It really does seem to work better if the non-breastfeeding partner does it.

- The £3.50 foldable Ikea 'sick bowl' earned its keep mere days after purchase, when the whole household was hit with a bug, cat included.

- Doddl cutlery for toddlers, which is so much easier for them to grasp and which dramatically sped up mealtimes.

- *On the Night You Were Born* by Nancy Tillman. One of our favourite books, but it wasn't until around this time that I could get to the end without stifling a sob. On discovering that she has a new one out, *Because You're Mine*, I was struck by this Amazon review: 'Gorgeous illustrations as always. The only problem is I can't get to the end without crying.' A children's author of rare talent.

- Washing-up liquid, the ultimate stain remover. I detest most housework, but for some reason get great satisfaction from stain removal. The only thing it wasn't able to remove was dried-on vomit stains on the baby's mattress, for which steam cleaning was required.

- *In the Night Garden*. 'Why is Makka Pakka half the size of Upsy Daisy, not to mention the enormous Igglepiggle?' asked my husband, who was less awed by it than the baby. 'Scale is a real issue in this programme. Look at the tiny Tombliboos.' 'No,' I said, 'it's the Pontipines that are really tiny. The Tombliboos are bigger than Makka Pakka but smaller than Igglepiggle.' Normal conversation will resume when my son reaches eighteen.

- *Sunstroke*, Tessa Hadley's short story collection. I was a long-time fan, but this time I read it from a new perspective, that of 'the warm vegetable soup of motherhood.' No one writes families better than Hadley.

- 'Why don't you look like a shoe?' my friend said, suspiciously, when she met me for lunch shortly after I gave birth. The reason? YSL's Touche Éclat concealer for making me look less haggard after all the sleepless nights, plus Beauty Pie's Superluminous Under-Eye Genius cream.

- Cheese as a vehicle for getting green veg into the baby. Like his mother, who is frequently mocked by his father for always adding it to dishes 'for flavour,' the baby is a *fromage* fiend, and will eat almost anything as long as it features. A friend uses a similar strategy, but with desiccated coconut. Yes, on everything, including bolognese.

What didn't

- Not having a dishwasher. Along with 'living up so many steps/stairs,' it was another thing to file under the category of 'should maybe have thought about this and rectified it before having a baby.'

- My work–life balance. The set-up of three days of stay-at-home mothering, two days of nursery, made me feel a bit Betty Draper. My son was a gorgeous age, but I wasn't a natural stay-at-home mother. Admitting this, and eventually switching to three days a week of nursery, made a big difference to my mental well-being, and therefore his.

- Hand, Foot and Mouth: a truly medieval disease. Thankfully, I managed to escape it, having had it as a child. Another parent told me darkly that their toenails fell off. As for the sores inside the mouth that made eating or drinking agony for my son, the following things helped: Anbesol liquid, ice cream, watermelon, yoghurt and chilled baby-food pouches.

- Postpartum friendships, apparently. I enjoyed an article in *New York* magazine, 'Why Can't Our Friendship Survive Your Baby?', about the impact a baby can have on friendship groups, although I didn't identify with it. What's changed, I think, is that more and more women are choosing to be childfree and feeling entitled to child-free time, whereas historically they would be roped into communal child-rearing. This is a reasonable expectation, but we all need to be kind to one another, and new parents are especially vulnerable. During this period, you need your friends more than ever, even if they're sick of hearing about it.

- Socks. At least the weather was getting better, so I wasn't getting so many dirty looks at the fact he was in bare feet.

- The biting phase. I spent this time having chunks bitten out of me, I think because my son was experiencing particularly bad teething pains. I was literally covered in little mouth-shaped bruises, and his key worker started wearing a puffer coat indoors.

- We unwittingly created a sleep association with Norah Jones's 2002 blockbuster album *Come Away With Me*, so our home environment now sounds like a Blairite dinner party. To this day, Spotify tells us we are in her top 1 per cent of listeners worldwide.
- Mouth smears. This kid loves wiping his mouth on everything that isn't a cloth. Feeding him turned into a race against time: can you wipe his grubby chops before he launches himself at your lovely blouse or the nearest piece of furniture? The answer is almost always no, which is why our furniture was covered in little rings of yoghurt.

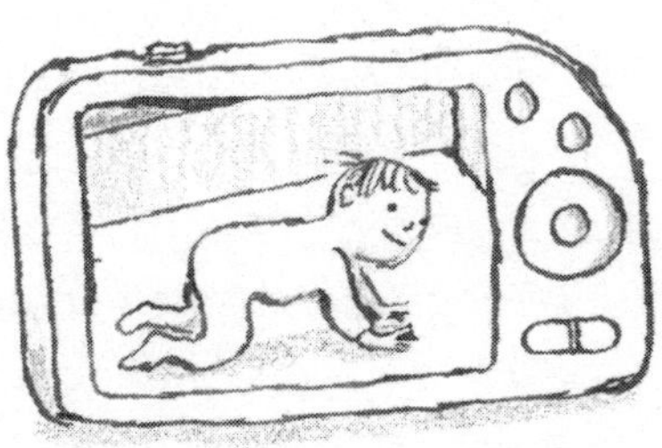

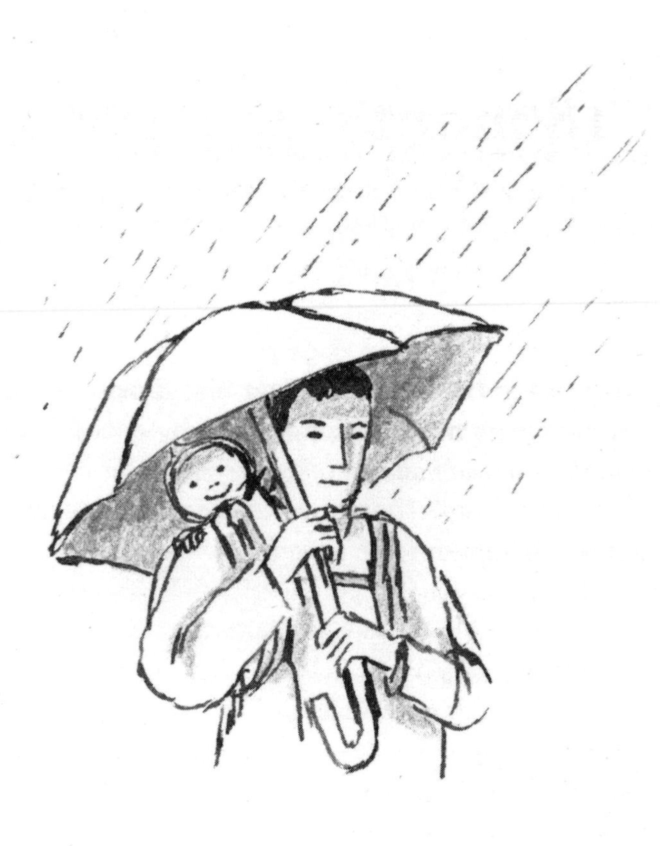

18 months to 2 years

My son's face lit up at Winnie-the-Pooh – and my misgivings melted away

(Or: On the powerful nostalgia of Disney)

Parenthood is replete with madeleines. Not just in the cake form – when I was struggling to breastfeed and trying to up my milk supply, I bought bags and bags of them, dipped in chocolate – but the famous Proustian kind. These small encounters with objects or sounds or smells act as nostalgic triggers, with the ability to catapult you back to moments in your childhood that you had long forgotten with a surprising emotional force.

It's perhaps less romantic when you discover that Proust initially wanted to use toast for his metaphor. Although, actually, I've always found toast to be hugely evocative. The sight of a schoolboy on a September morning cradling a slice in a sheet of kitchen roll reminded me recently of how my mother – along with, I suspect, mothers everywhere – used to thrust toast into my hands as I rushed out of the door, late for the bus.

Then, this week, another madeleine, this time in the form of Disney. More specifically, the intro: the flag, the fireworks, the screen panning out to show the pitched turrets of the castle.

The strings playing 'When You Wish Upon a Star'. My God. I had forgotten all about it, but in a split second I was four again, lying on the floor of the living room in our little terraced house in Chorlton, Manchester, with the lights out and all the curtains closed and the VHS of *The Jungle Book* starting up for the fifteenth time that week. Years of ambivalence towards, and at times even discomfort with, the Disney corporation swept away in one fell swoop, compounded by the look of sheer, transfixed delight on my child's face as he watched Winnie-the-Pooh singing about honey. Take my money, Disney, take it all!

Disney is, of course, powered by this kind of adult nostalgia. It is part of its modus operandi, and central to its profit motive. I'm also aware that 'Disney adults' – as grown-ups who really, really love Disney are termed – are widely disdained, to the point that they have been called 'the most hated group on the internet'. The studio turns 100 this year, and has released a short film containing a plethora of characters new and old in celebration, many of which I recognised from my own childhood viewing. Yet it left me fairly cold.

Though I was raised on Disney fairy tales, my mother always made sure that its more saccharine, gendered, princess output (of which I was a faithful acolyte) was counterbalanced with feminist alternatives. Then, when I grew up, I read *From the Beast to the Blonde* and *The Bloody Chamber*. So I'm very aware of the Disneyfication of traditional fairy tales and the gender stereotyping that (particularly older) Disney princess films peddle, while recognising that little girls are probably better off watching a *Sleeping Beauty* that doesn't contain rape and cannibalism, even if she does have a 22in waist. (Incidentally, I was bemused to hear rumours that Disney will be adapting *Bluebeard*. Just how, exactly, do you manage to put a happy Disney filter on that tale of imprisonment and decapitation?)

That's before you get to the racial stereotyping, from *Dumbo* to *Aladdin*, and *Song of the South* – a film so racist that Disney has prevented its release on any home video or streaming platform, but I'm old enough to remember 'Zip-a-Dee-Doo-Dah' playing at the end of other features as part of a Disney singalong. I'm not about to start donning a pair of Minnie Mouse ears in the queue for the 'It's a Small World' ride, let's put it that way.

That doesn't mean that I'm immune, though, now that I have my own small boy whose face lights up at the sight of Christopher Robin. This is potent stuff, and I won't be the last parent willing to overlook their principles because of something that makes their child happy. In fact, I've been fairly laissez-faire about lots of things you might expect a *Guardian* columnist to get annoyed about, from ultra-processed melty puffs to screen time. Everyone has their own red lines in parenthood. Mine happen to be toy guns and kids' clothes with slogans on them. But Disney? There has been much improvement in recent years in terms of representation, and I genuinely enjoyed watching *Mary Poppins Returns* at Christmas, even tearing up about the poor, bereaved Banks children. (Disney has never shied away from death – like many of his generation, my father remembers having to be taken, traumatised, out of *Bambi*.)

One of the questions new parents seem to ask a lot is, 'When does it get easier?' A friend with a newborn recently said she's looking forward to this, and I avoided telling her that I found six to twelve months even harder than the first bit. But another friend reassuringly puts a marker on it; it gets easier, she says, when they'll sit through a whole Disney feature and you can go about your business. That is, of course, if you don't spend the whole film mooning over their smile.

I feared my mental health struggles would hold my son back, but I'm starting to see they could help him

(Or: In which I am having a very hard time)

I've been having a tough time with my mental health lately. Anxiety and low mood have been compounded by my son's repeated night wakings, and after settling him I have been lying wide awake, heart racing with adrenaline. Averaging three hours of sleep a night, it was inevitable that I would burn out with exhaustion eventually, requiring time off work.

Just typing these words, and the thought of you reading them, makes me feel shame. Shame that I haven't coped better, shame at the burden it has placed on others, and shame that I'm feeling this way, when, considering the pain and trauma others are facing, I am lucky. That feeling of shame always creates in me an impulse to write. When I first started this series, mere weeks after giving birth, a female journalist I have known for years suggested that I was too vulnerable to be doing so. Yet if we never create work from a place of vulnerability, I am not sure what writing is for.

It is hard to accept feeling vulnerable as a parent. You are supposed to be strong for the small human(s) you are caring for, and so being confronted with the notion that you might fall apart and therefore let them down only adds to feelings of despair and self-disgust. It's no secret that I've struggled with my mental health in the past; I have written about it in this newspaper, and my memoir, *The Year of the Cat*, is partly about how you make the decision to have a baby – with all the fear that can entail – when you have a history of anxiety, in my case post-traumatic stress disorder (PTSD). There are those who argue that it's fairer not to reproduce, and I have been moved by friends' and readers' experiences of how it can feel to grow up with a parent who isn't coping. In my lower moments this past month I have been haunted by the character of the chronically depressed mum in *About a Boy*, and the impact that her mental illness has on her unhappy son, Marcus.

On the other hand, one in four of us experience some form of mental health issue in any given year, and as with other medical conditions and disabilities, implying that such people should never become parents is deeply ableist. Some of the best parents I know are those who have lived with anxiety and depression, and they have been inspirational in my decision to become a mother.

I have been lucky in that I received support, first from an NHS psychology service specialising in women's health, and then from the perinatal mental health team. I didn't write about it at the time, because I didn't know how to. I was quite rightly discharged after we concluded that I – thankfully – wasn't suffering from a perinatal mental illness, but I credit the extra support, especially in the early months, with the fact that I was able to cope so well with a difficult premature birth and early motherhood. If only all new parents could access such help.

Becoming a parent involves seismic life and hormonal changes, and can awaken in us feelings about our childhoods and family relationships of which we may not have been previously aware. Suddenly you see the way that you were parented – for good and for bad – through new eyes. Your relationships – with your partner, your friends – often shift, as does the way you think about work. In other words, it's a lot, before you even consider the effects of sleeplessness.

A mental health nurse told me that the best thing for anyone suffering from mental illness is sleep, which is of course mostly off limits to new parents. Until I became a parent, I had never really thought about how lack of sleep is just taken as a given, how you are just supposed to get on with it, despite everyone wryly commenting that it's used as a method of torture. We know that people feel their lowest between 4 a.m. and 5 a.m. – during the darkness before the dawn, as I try to remember to think of it – and I have been awake far too often during these hours in recent weeks. Even when my husband took on the nights, which he has done over and over again, I would lie there awake in the next room with an inner anxiety monologue that would not stop.

I'm not better, but I'm in a better place. Little things have helped – seeing my son happy, which he is, despite this tough patch of mine. When I blow bubbles, he and the cat congregate and compete to pop them, which is just so joyful. My husband offers unwavering love and support, as do my friends and family. One friend, a masseuse, gave me a free massage. Another gave me some CBD oil, which now has me sleeping like a log even between wakings. A third took me out for a wonderful lunch. A fourth came to the playground and we ate cannoli and drank coffee while we pushed the baby on the swing. The past few weeks have confirmed for me that we have not evolved to parent in such small units: humans need people.

I'll be getting more therapy, in the hope that it can help prevent me burning out again, but I've already been trying to put what I've learned from therapists in the past into practice to make it easier to cope. Practising gratitude has been so helpful because it is not just about reflecting on the good things in your life, but it actively rewires your brain so that you become more attuned to the positives around you. Lying there in the dark, in despair, I found myself focusing on the fact that my family and I are safe, warm in our beds, while other parents and children, particularly those in Gaza, one of the most densely child-populated places in the world, are not so fortunate. A friend who is a GP always says that it's good to be grateful, but it's also OK to say you're having a shit time. Maintaining perspective, however, and feeling empathy for others, can be a galvanising force; a reminder to focus on solidarity and hope.

Instead of causing us shame, hard times can teach us things. I am coming to understand that my struggles, rather than holding my son back, will allow me to pass on to him some of the tools to weather life's storms.

I resist sharenting on social media. Does that mean my son and I are missing out, or is it just safer?

(Or: On keeping your child's face off the internet)

An old friend asked me recently why I never put my son's face online. 'Can you explain the not showing pics of babies thing to me?' she asked. 'Everyone our age seems to obscure their baby's face with emojis. I feel as if I've missed a key essay on the morality of baby pic social media publication.'

I don't do the emoji thing – in fact I've even stopped showing the back of his head, or any aspect of his home life, really – but I know what she means. A few years ago, sharenting, as it's been called, felt like the norm among my social circle. These days I see far fewer babies' faces on social media. Concerns about online privacy and safeguarding, as well as facial recognition and the commercial use of personal data, are far more prevalent than they were in the early days of Facebook. In fact, you could say that whether or not you share photos has become another parental identity marker, up there with breastfeeding, cloth nappies and baby-led weaning as evidence that you're doing things 'the right way', not like 'those other parents'.

I have my own reasons for not publishing photos of my child, relating to my job as a female writer with a modest public profile, so I'm not sure how relevant my views on it are to other parents. If I'm honest, I have always felt that there was something dystopian about putting a child's life online without their consent. In fact, one of the pieces that got me this job was a student newspaper column I wrote back in 2011, which envisaged every significant moment of a child's life, from conception to grave, mediated through the spectacle of social media.

This didn't stop me hypocritically wanting to share photographs of myself with friends' babies, however, and once I became a mother the temptation to show him off has been strong. So I understand both sides of the argument, and also recognise that these decisions are often in flux. Many parents, for instance, might stop sharing once their bald little infants start to look more like identifiable people. Others, having learned about online safeguarding, have gone back and deleted photos, or won't post anything that could be used nefariously by paedophiles. Lots of parents lock down their social media accounts, keeping their small followings to people that they know in real life, and regularly pruning their friend lists.

When I asked people to share their views, the parents who were most cautious were those who, like me, have jobs that might render their children more vulnerable to being recognised: criminal barristers, NHS staff working in mental health, anyone with a public profile. 'Our lives aren't less because of it,' one mum says. 'I work in HR and I like my life private, and when she's older I can tell her I kept her life private until she has her own social media if she chooses.' Another, who has worked on online safety in schools, is concerned about identity theft. 'It terrifies me how many people will share on social media their child's name and date of birth and then use the latter as a password for their bank account. Doctors just ask for name and DOB for security, schools and nurseries often use middle names as passwords for collection … A lifetime of being told not to share personal information with strangers, and I could tell you the full names, birthdays, places of birth and schools of ten people I know on social media but not in real life.'

As with many aspects of parenthood, I think the question of online sharing also boils down to: just how anxious are you? One mother, who loves seeing and sharing cute baby photos, says she has what she calls a 'naturally high fear threshold', so just as she defiantly walks alone at night, she feels that the joy and community of sharing photographs with other parents outweighs the risks. 'I feel that so much of being a parent is marred by fear and I think that this is also leading children to grow up in an unhealthily fearful environment,' another mother tells me. Parenting can be isolating, especially when you live away from family, and many of the parents who got in touch to say they happily share photos of their children do so for that reason. 'They are a part of you, and it's difficult to share your life without them in it,' says a friend, who before having her son had been adamant she wouldn't share pictures of him but now does. 'He's most of my social life at the moment and it's an easy way to feel connected to this network of people who love him that doesn't involve me writing hundreds of individual messages,' says another. Others tell me that sharing their experience of pregnancy loss helped them get through it, and sharing the positive outcome of that awful time – a much-wanted baby – has been a continuation of that openness.

Even if you don't want your child's face online, negotiating with grandparents and other relatives can be tricky. Perhaps surprisingly, the older generation often seem less fazed about online security than their offspring, with grandparents desperate to show pictures on Facebook and some even going against the wishes of the parents. Discussing these boundaries can be fraught at times, and it often seems to be women who feel the most pressure to share. This makes sense, considering research has found that women are frequently absent from family photographs because it is they who 'manage the family heritage, who take the photos, classify them, comment on them and share them'.

A primary school teacher who contacted me said that every year, she hears children complaining about the amount their parents share about them online. For me, and many other parents, it comes down to consent. I'd like my son to negotiate his digital footprint on his terms, but I understand and respect that other parents feel differently, and also wonder if the children without any digital footprint might wonder why, or feel left out. Ultimately, whatever we decide, it's worth remembering that one day, we might have to sit down with our children and explain our reasoning.

I want my son to wear fun, colourful clothes – but boys' fashion is so boring

(Or: On the tyranny of trucks)

For my sins, I went to Primark this week. I usually try to avoid the high street for ethical reasons, but occasionally I have to buy the bairn some socks. He has a penchant for shedding them all over north London, and he finds shoes highly offensive, and it has been costing me a fortune. As I navigated the sea of pink and sparkle that is the girls' section, I found myself looking at rack after rack of blue and grey boys' trousers, and wondering yet again, why so many clothes for little boys are just so bloody boring.

When garments aren't plain or muted, they are covered in trucks, robots or dinosaurs. I'm fine with dinosaurs (how can you not be?) but I refuse to buy him anything with trucks on it, or worse, diggers. I don't even really understand what heavy plant machinery has to do with children, who are quite rightly forbidden from its operation. Also off the table are the ubiquitous beefeaters (the boy is part-Welsh and the only approved monarch under our roof was murdered by the English in 1282); most slogans, on account of them being naff and/or nonsensical; superheroes; the police; farmyard animals with the exception of sheep; and the Gruffalo, who, let's be honest, is no oil painting.

Now, before you start furiously composing an email to me with a subject line containing the words 'tofu-eating wokerati', this isn't just about gender politics, although that is an aspect of it. It's also personal taste. I have always loved and had strong opinions about clothes, and dressing up should be fun, especially for children and especially for boys. I can't help feeling that they get a raw deal when compared with little girls.

So much more imagination seems to go into clothing design for the latter, notwithstanding the tyranny of pink, weirdly sexy cuts and 'be kind' slogans.

I'd have known where I was, clothes-wise, with a girl, what with me being one. Of course, you can dress your child in a completely gender-neutral way. I found out my son was a son when I met him for the first time and my husband said, his voice catching, 'It's our boy.' I'd had my suspicions before that, after my husband thought he saw 'something' on the 20-week scan, although he said: 'It could have been a leg, I didn't know what I was looking at.' As such, my son's first clothes were gender-neutral hand-me-downs from his little friend Zayley.

I do quite like pretty dresses and would undoubtedly have put a daughter in them. My own mother used to make a lot of my clothes and seemed to enjoy dressing me up like a small Edwardian, with lovely floral dresses and lace petticoats, accessorised with lace-up boots or a straw hat. I'm progressive and a feminist, but I wasn't about to put my son in bloomers. So what to do?

My French aunt set the tone with some beautiful, vibrant gifts from Petit Bateau. I was once sacked from a nannying job for not ironing some Petit Bateau polo necks on the correct setting, but I seem to have finally processed that trauma. Hand-me-downs from his cousin were also fabulous. I decided to do some research. I looked on Instagram. I looked at the other babies at the stay-and-play and asked their parents where they got their stuff. I looked at what the children of celebrities wore, at one point falling into a Prince George rabbit hole before exiting largely unconvinced but nonetheless having bought a sailor suit. I googled fun children's clothing brands and found that lack of imagination on the mainstream British high street is cast into even sharper relief when you look at the wonderful kids' clothes that continental and small sustainable brands are producing. But these clothes are often more expensive, which is how I discovered Vinted.

What would parents do without Vinted, where for a couple of quid you can pick up an almost-new Mini Boden jumper, a pair of Frugi parsnip pants, or a Bobo Choses bodysuit (I am obsessed with Bobo Choses, whose arty, brightly coloured clothes are just so joyful) that would normally cost £45? It has completely transformed the way parents shop, enabling us to buy directly from other parents in an affordable, ethical way. Its algorithm has given me so many ideas and has helped me find new clothing companies. As my son drifts off to sleep, I sit next to his crib scrolling and liking and making offers, dreaming up new outfit ideas for him. It makes me happy to kit him out and see him looking so sweet. I never thought I'd have so much fun dressing a boy.

I think my son looks great and so, it seems, do other people. It makes them smile and he gets a lot of compliments. His leopard-print tracksuit bottoms might raise eyebrows in some parts of the world, but not where I live. Here, people love a baby boy in a rainbow-coloured, hand-knitted cardigan, or a dungaree-and-top combination in clashing prints. I always try to make him look fun and joyful, but never ridiculous. He is occasionally mistaken for a girl, but mostly by people who think you have to put a bow on a baby girl's head so everyone can tell her sex. Mostly, people ask who he's wearing, like he's on the red carpet at the Met Gala. I have a list of favourite brands ready in response.

No doubt there are readers who will think it shallow that I've devoted so much time to my son's wardrobe. But I suspect they would be less judgmental if I did the same for a daughter. I hope that, in reading this, other parents will feel inspired and convinced that boys' clothes needn't be boring. After all, we only have a very short window in which to dress them before they are able to choose themselves. And if there comes a point where he decides he wants a T-shirt with the Gruffalo driving a digger on it, well, so be it.

My advice about the stress zone that is toddler mealtimes: do your best and get by – everything else is just noise

(Or: On maintaining your sanity when it comes to cooking)

Were I to pitch a cookbook, it would be this: healthy, easy toddler meals that take less than twenty minutes, for busy, tired parents who can't be arsed. It wouldn't be shiny or contain aspirational photographs of me, smiling with all my teeth as I one-handedly stir a laborious risotto while clutching a cherubic, catalogue-perfect baby, alongside scaremongery copy about baby-food pouches. No, it would be written in bullet points of a paragraph or less, with no frills at all. The recipes would read like this:

> Haddock risotto: 1) Boil egg. 2) Dot frozen haddock fillet with butter; microwave for $2\frac{1}{2}$ mins. 3) Microwave $\frac{1}{3}$ pack basmati rice for $1\frac{1}{2}$ mins. 4) Microwave peas with water for 4 mins. 5) Make cheese sauce. 6) Mix it all together.

It would also contain the sort of politically incorrect tips for getting your child to eat that would have the baby food influencers of Instagram phoning social services. Tips such as: put *Postman Pat* on and try again (thanks, mother-in-law!), mix in an Ella's Kitchen food pouch with the food they're refusing (sister-in-law), and add butter to the puree (a reader to whom I owe many peaceful nights).

I don't think it would sell much, because anyone who values their sanity is already doing some version of these things. Mealtimes with toddlers are stressful enough. The rise of the microwave – and therefore obesity – is often blamed on feminism. All those busy working mothers who stopped putting their families first by sweating over a stove for hours! But a microwave doesn't necessarily mean ready meals, as anyone who has looked at a 1970s microwave cookbook will tell you. You can make a surprising number of things in a microwave (whole sides of salmon! – the mind boggles). When a friend with two young children said she didn't have one, I asked her – once I had stopped screaming – how she survived. Every couple of months I make a slow-cook tomato and basil sauce and freeze the lot for defrosting in the microwave, and that has genuinely saved me.

I'm a bad mother, probably, because current parenting fashion dictates that I'm supposed to be feeding my boy exactly what we eat, instead of yesterday's reheated pasta from the pub. Often I do, but last night we had samphire because I fancied something extremely high in sodium, just as sometimes you want a curry that can blow your head off, not another creamy baby one.

Sometimes, also, I would like to eat dinner at a normal hour. Frequently, that bit in *Seinfeld* about the early bird special pops into my mind ('It's 4:30.' 'Who eats dinner at 4:30?' 'By the time we sit down it'll be quarter to five.'). I would also like time in which to eat it. My book would include a whole section on indigestion, and also tips on how to maximise cooking for your family as the only break you'll get that day (wine, Bruce Springsteen).

Here in north London, my husband and I make most of our meals from scratch, but I still find other parents quite judgy. My Welsh friends don't seem to have as many hang-ups about feeding their babies ready-made banana porridge. Just the other day, another mother told me, in horrified tones, that her parents used to just blitz up whatever they were eating for dinner and feed it to them. Her baby was gummily mouthing a radicchio leaf at the time, but I couldn't work out what the problem was. You mean you don't just put the chicken cacciatore in the blender? Doesn't everyone do that?

I had obviously forgotten about the baby-led-weaning orthodoxy, having blanked the annoying weaning months from my memory (I hated being made to feel that I was a bad mother for not making veggie muffins). I spoon-fed my child and, despite my being told this would make him a picky eater, he will now eat anything, even things I couldn't stomach until I was an adult: olives, anchovies and baba ganoush with so much garlic it walked before he did. And now that he eats anything, the time spent making muffins feels more worth it. There is great pleasure to be had in watching your child enjoy something you've lovingly prepared.

I'm not smug, though, because I know that there will come a day when he will only want chicken nuggets and chips, and it will be absolutely no reflection on me. It's normal to link your identity to food – it says so much about who we are, our culture and our values – but when it comes to parenting, the competitiveness can be next level. It all just seems so pointless, when you can do everything by the book and still end up with a picky eater. Children are very much themselves, and if they don't want to eat the sweet potato falafel, they are not going to eat it; people who boast 'mine eat what they're given or they'll starve' fail to understand this.

You have to do what you can to get by, and everything else is just noise. Mealtimes can be taxing enough without looking at other parents askance for how they choose to do it. My brother is autistic and never liked sitting at the table. Instead of forcing him, my mother simply let him wander in and out, picking at what he wanted on the plate. Why make life more difficult for everyone?

My toddler is going through a phase of being very suspicious of the first mouthful of any food he is presented with, as though he is a medieval king who has heard rumours of a poisoning plot. I, his lowly jester, must therefore perform the dance of the seven spoons, which involves trying to put the spoon in his mouth (he still loves to be fed – my fault for not doing BLW) while he knocks it out of my hand. I get another spoon. He flails wildly until the exact moment when the food touches his lips, at which point he waves it in like he's an air traffic controller. Mmm yes, more of that. It's a fun game for us both. No doubt there will be many more fun games to come, which is why there would also be a chapter on stain removal.

Ten lazy person's toddler meals that take fifteen minutes or less

1 Deconstructed fish pie

- Put a salmon fillet in the oven (15 mins) or if you're really lazy, you can use frozen fillets which microwave in less than 5 minutes, but don't have as nice a texture.
- Put some new potatoes on to boil (15 mins) or microwave for 3 minutes.
- When salmon and potatoes are nearly ready, put some frozen peas in the microwave.
- Make a parsley sauce, or – laziest of all – heat some crème fraiche on the hob with a bit of whole milk. Add parsley.
- Mash potatoes with some butter using a fork, flake the salmon, serve the peas, drizzle with sauce.

2 Cheesy scrambled eggs

- Grate cheese into eggs while scrambling. Serve with toast and avocado.

3 Baked sweet potato with broccoli cheese filling

- Microwave a sweet potato (about 5 minutes depending on size).
- Cook some frozen broccoli, either on the hob or in a saucepan until it's soft enough (4 or 5 minutes). Drain and chop it up small.
- Return the broccoli to a saucepan and, on a low heat, add some ricotta or cream cheese until it starts to melt. Add a splash of whole milk, and, if desired, some cheddar.
- Slice sweet potato and spread it with butter. Top it with the broccoli cheese. (The broccoli cheese also makes an easy pasta sauce.)

4 Lentil bolognese

- Put some pasta on to boil.
- Heat some oil and fry chopped celery, carrot and onion until soft (about 6 minutes). Add minced garlic and fry for a minute. Add whichever herbs you like – I tend to use dried mixed herbs.
- Add a tin of green lentils.
- Add a tin of chopped tomatoes/plum tomatoes/passata and heat until sauce is bubbling and the carrots are fully soft. Serve with fresh basil and grated cheese.
- (For an equally quick deconstructed lentil shepherd's pie, simply add a small amount of flour after the garlic and herbs, cook for 1 minute before adding the lentils, a splash of low-salt stock and a squirt of tomato puree instead of the canned tomatoes, and serve it with mashed potato or sweet potato)

5 Sweet potato quesadillas

- Microwave a sweet potato.
- Scoop it out and combine the flesh with butter and a splash of milk, mashing with a fork.
- Spread it on a tortilla wrap and sprinkle with grated cheese and some paprika.
- Place another wrap on top and press down. Fry for a minute or two on each side. Cut into triangles, and serve with mashed avocado.

6 Mac and peas

- Boil macaroni.
- Cook frozen peas in the microwave. Retain a small amount of the water and blitz with ricotta or cream cheese until it's a smooth sauce.
- Mix in the cooked pasta.

7 Butternut risotto

(I prefer to use a pre-boiled wheat grain called Ebly for this, but it would also work with microwave rice, couscous, quick-cook spelt, or orzo).

- Prepare your grain of choice.
- Cut up a butternut squash, or, if you really can't be arsed, you can buy it cubed and/or frozen.
- Boil for 5 minutes until soft. Towards the end add a couple of handfuls of spinach.
- Meanwhile, fry an onion. If you like, you can add some chopped mushrooms and fry for a few minutes until soft. Add minced garlic and dried herbs.
- Add the grains. Drain the butternut and spinach, retaining a splash of the water. Mix the butternut and spinach and water in with the other ingredients until the butternut starts to fall apart.
- Add whichever cheese you like. It works well with goat's cheese, or parmesan.

8 Dad's veggie rice

This is my husband's recipe for using up whatever leftover veg is in the fridge, plus some store cupboard staples. He experiments with different kinds of bean, but black-eyed, black beans or kidney beans work well.

- Fry a chopped onion. Add chopped vegetables of your choice, such as leek, courgettes, peppers, carrots, etc.
- Add spices of your choice – we use paprika, cumin and mild chilli, as well as garlic. Put in a big squirt of tomato puree.
- Fry until soft, then stir in a packet of microwave rice, a tin of beans, and sweetcorn if you choose to use it.
- Serve with a fried egg on top, chopped herbs and a squeeze of lime juice, and hot sauce for the adults.

9 Chickpea curry

- Fry a chopped onion. When it is starting to soften, add minced garlic (you can buy it in a jar either on its own or mixed with ginger from Asian supermarkets if you prefer) and grated ginger.
- Add your spices of choice. When we were starting him on solids we tended to avoid chilli powder, but we'd use cumin, coriander, turmeric, etc. If you're not confident with spices, you could use a mild curry powder or garam masala, or a paste. Stir it all together for a minute or two.
- Add a can of chopped tomatoes and a can of chickpeas.
- Simmer for 5 or 6 minutes.
- Add a handful or two of spinach and cook for two more minutes.
- If you like, stir in crème fraiche, yoghurt or coconut milk.
- Serve with microwave rice and chopped coriander.

10 Ham carbonara

I started making this when I was being more cautious about salt. Now that he's older, I tend to make carbonara the conventional way, with guanciale or pancetta, and just limit how much meat he gets in his bowl.

- Boil dried pasta, or even faster – fresh tagliatelle.
- While the pasta is cooking, chop and fry some ham in butter until it's crispy. Add as much garlic as you choose and fry for a minute.
- In a large mixing bowl, crack at least two eggs (depending on how many people are eating, you can add more if you like) and mix them with a handful of grated parmesan, pecorino or – if you must, but don't tell any Italians – cheddar. Add pepper.
- Conserve a ladle or two of pasta water and drain the pasta. Tip it into the frying pan with the ham. Mix well.

- Add the pasta and ham to the mixing bowl and, stirring quickly, mix well, adding pasta water to get the desired consistency. As long as you keep tossing it, the hot pasta cooks the egg without scrambling it. (NB. Always use British Lion eggs!)

This was the year I nearly resorted to an elite baby sleep trainer. But there is another way

(Or: On how my husband saved my sanity)

Sleep, I came to understand this year, is everything. Without sleep, action, change and momentum all feel impossible. Without sleep, you are living half a life, an existence that is less about living and more about getting through. My husband and I entered 2023 in a state of complete exhaustion. Our baby had been hospitalised several times and through a combination of terror, survival and necessity, he and I had entered a co-sleeping arrangement that saw him waking every hour for milk.

My husband was working full time and I was trying to juggle being essentially a stay-at-home mother with writing my column and promoting a book. The only reason I was still sane was because my husband consistently shared feeding and nights from the beginning, and at the worst times would often take the baby until the early hours so I could get a block of sleep from, say, 8 p.m. until 2 a.m. If I had had a less supportive husband or a baby that didn't take a bottle from him, or if my lovely mother hadn't stepped in when things got really tough, I suspect I would have lost my mind.

We didn't sleep-train – we hadn't needed to. We were those people whose baby slept through from eight weeks, blissful on his back in a starfish position – the ones who stay quiet when other parents despair of the frequent night wakings and strategise solutions with each other. We never talked about it unless we were directly asked, 'How is he sleeping?' Just wait for the four-month sleep regression, people said, darkly. But that never came. How smug we were, how self-satisfied at our infant's ability to self-settle, the fact that he instinctively seemed to know how to tank up before bed.

What fools.

It was illness that did for our baby's sleep. He came to rely on the comfort and reassurance of milk and touch, and we refused to deprive him of it, despite it being repeatedly suggested that we sleep-train. I have never judged those who do; a mum who has let a baby cry it out is better than a dead mum (and I have friends who were so exhausted that they started to wish themselves away). But it wasn't for me. I knew I would crack. His sobs cut through me like a knife.

Which is how I came to hear of Brenda Hart. 'You should get Nanny Brenda,' another mother said to me in the playground, her voice slightly lowered as if to acknowledge that her suggestion crossed a Rubicon. I live in Islington, surrounded by rich people who can afford to throw money at their problems, so this was not the first time I had heard the name of the elite sleep trainer. I'd even read about her in the *New Yorker*, where Sam Knight described her as 'a matron of the old school'. Her method is simple: you shut the door and let the baby cry it out.

Despite my previous resolve not to do this, I started fantasising about hiring Brenda, not caring by this point how much it cost. I went back and forth endlessly in a way that she would probably roll her eyes at. I observed the sleep training wars of Mumsnet, internalising all the worst messages: leaving him to cry even for a minute would damage him irrevocably. A chastising paragraph from Philippa Perry's *The Book You Wish Your Parents Had Read*, which paid no heed at all to maternal mental health in its discussion of sleep training, haunted me. I believed on some level that sleep training would make me a bad mother. Yet I desperately needed rest. All I could think about and talk about was sleep.

You're probably wondering, 'Where's the hope?' Did it lie with Nanny Brenda? Though Hart's success is undeniable, we didn't hire her in the end.

Several things happened to change our lives. A perinatal psychologist recommended a book called *Through the Night: Helping Parents and Sleepless Infants* by Dilys Daws, which is based on the idea that one should listen to the 'cries' of the family as a whole. She says that when our baby cries, we hear ourselves crying as a baby, and our thoughts and feelings about how to respond are shaped by our own early experiences. That book, as well as my therapist, helped me understand that I feared separation would make my child anxious later in life, when in fact by failing to separate I could unwittingly be giving him the message that the world was unsafe without me there. Turning my fear on its head this way was truly transformative.

Also, the baby started nursery, and was more tuckered out and had a more structured nap routine. But most importantly, I emailed Sam Knight at the *New Yorker*, who suggested that before hiring Brenda, we give his own, gentler method a try. 'Keep going!' he signed off. 'This too will pass.' Hope!

I read Sam's emails to my husband and we devised a plan for him to night-wean the baby (it has to be the man that does it, because the baby can smell its mother's milk). My husband took a week off work, and each night he picked the baby up every time he cried, cuddled him until he was calm, and put him down. The first night he must have done this thirty times. The second, ten. The third, three. On the fourth night, my son slept through. Life was transformed, and largely thanks to two dads: Sam Knight and my lovely husband, who pushed himself to the limit for our family. (Perhaps they should go into business, charging £500 a pop.) I am beyond thankful to them both.

I'm not saying that sleep is ever perfect, but I'm writing this to pass on the hope. To those parents who are reading this in a similarly dark place, keep going: sleep can be yours again.

What worked

- My son, who took his first steps at a corrected age of seventeen months, was by age two walking confidently and steadily, though I was secretly pleased that he still wanted to hold my hand rather than running off over the horizon. I was and am so proud of him.

- This easy pizza dough recipe courtesy of Organix (250g self-raising flour/plain flour with 3 tsp. baking powder; 4 tbsp olive oil; 100ml warm water) is fantastic.

- We switched to a duvet and a quilt, and got better sleep as a result. I was bowled over by the sheer intricacy, imagination and skill that has gone into the bedding created by Rebecca Monserat and Alice Ruby Ross, whose small sustainable British business, Forivor, aims to foster in children an early love of nature. These heirloom products are like living storybooks, and I actually gasped when opening the parcel. I'm a thrifty shopper, but to my mind the beauty of the design justifies the price, and they make lovely gifts.

- The humidifier. Since the previous winter's awful bout of bronchiolitis, which saw my son hospitalised several times, every virus went straight to his chest. With eucalyptus oil, the humidifier was able to calm his cough enough for him to get to sleep and – miracles of miracles – he slept through the night.

- The music of Vicky Arlidge, who I discovered when looking for nursery rhymes on Spotify that were sung in a British accent. She has a lovely voice and her renditions have a folky, traditional style, which means they are much more pleasant for adults. My son loves drifting off to sleep to them.

- Baby disco! My son got some disco lights for Christmas and now most evenings before bed we have a dance in the living room. He loves music and it burns off his residual energy, but the best thing is looking at his smiling face when I spin him around the room. It's become our special time, and he gave me such a lovely spontaneous kiss and cuddle the other day that, like the sap that I am, I burst into tears during Katy Perry's 'Firework.'
- Picard frozen organic creamed spinach. The bairn loves it, and it microwaves in minutes. It's not cheap, but a little goes a really long way, and it makes a really quick pasta sauce.

What didn't

- Tantrums. We started seeing some signs of toddler tantrums. He didn't want to sit in his high chair, or get out of the swing, or go in the bath. I suspected he knew what he was doing; there's a page of the book *My Big Shouting Day!* by Rebecca Patterson where the little girl rolls around the floor yelling 'NO BED NO NO NO NO BED NO NO!' He thought it was absolutely hilarious.
- The Beatles. The bairn loves to dance, and you'd think tiring him out would mean an early bedtime, but the other night he danced to fifteen Beatles No. 1 singles in a row and was wide awake as ever.

- I love reading to my son, and he loves the sound of rhymes, but I am still annoyed by how many children's books contain lines that simply don't scan. Call me a pedant, but it should be a condition of publication that the book is read aloud first, and that any clunky, crammed-in extra syllables are revised.

- The weather. Never is the absence of places to go with a toddler more apparent than during days when the rain is pouring down and your child is stuck inside climbing the walls. I can't work out why there aren't more parent-friendly cafe's with playrooms. The ones we've been to are great and seem to be thriving, so there's clearly a market there.

- The Elf on the Shelf. A friend failed to consider that her three-year-old might be alarmed at the prospect of a toy becoming sentient at night. Her daughter was highly concerned and insisted on laying down some ground rules. 'Dear Elf,' their letter reads, 'Here are some rules. You are not allowed to scare me. You have to stay downstairs and not come to my room. Also, don't touch me.' 'I'm considering just burning the thing ceremonially,' my friend says.

- 'Gentle parenting.' We were only at the beginning of the toddler tantrum phase, and thankfully at this age our boy was still easily distracted and comforted (but how long will that last?). I've seen enough well-meaning parents trying to negotiate with children melting down on pavements to be a bit sceptical about the trend, and there seems to be a backlash happening from people who fear we are raising a generation of kids that have never heard the word 'no.'

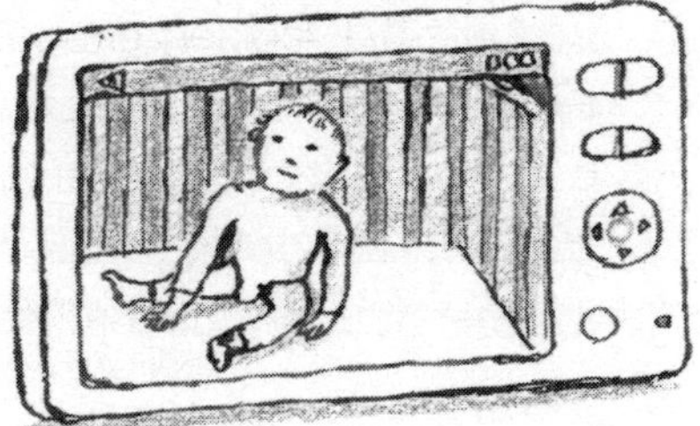

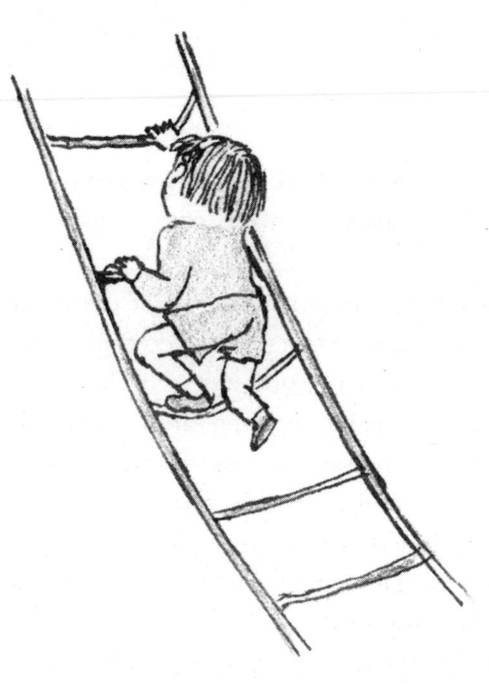

Parenthood is Political

Whether you're 'childless' or 'childfree', you shouldn't have to talk about it

In recent years, I've heard members of the older generation complain that it is no longer considered acceptable to ask a younger person whether or not they have children. It's true that this isn't polite, especially during small talk with a stranger. They may as well be saying: 'So, tell me all about the inner workings of your/your partner's uterus.'

Personally, I used to dread this question, even more so when it was framed as, 'Do you have a family?' Of course I do, I just haven't birthed any of them. People's feelings on procreation are often complicated, sometimes painful, and always deeply personal. In the context of increasing panic about the birth rate, the question of having children – or not, as it may be – is even more loaded, because it intersects with so many other factors in our lives: health, finances, employment status, gender or sexuality, housing, relationship status and so on. These are not things you necessarily want to delve into over the course of a casual conversation.

Or, perhaps – revolutionary as it might sound – you simply don't want to have children, and it's your right to not want to discuss that or be interrogated about that.

The fact that the word 'childless' seems to be going out of fashion is largely to be celebrated. It positions having a child as the default, and has the power to be intensely wounding. As a word, it carries with it a feeling of 'lacking', when that is certainly not everyone's experience. This stigma is why the term 'childfree' is increasingly becoming the default in media reporting after being popularised on internet message boards in recent years.

I was interested in how people without children may feel about that, so I've been asking them on- and offline whether they see the use of 'childfree' as an improvement. People who had chosen not to have children generally preferred to be referred to as 'childfree', but those whose 'childlessness' was involuntary, due to infertility, bereavement or life circumstances, felt erased by it. Many complained that both terms positioned having children as the default, when it shouldn't be ('I'm just a woman living life,' said one respondent). Why define by deficit? Indeed, I'd say the overwhelming majority disliked both words, with one being seen as stigmatising and the other gleeful and nasty in its implication that parents somehow need 'liberating'.

Others took issue with the term 'childfree' because it has become the chosen moniker for an online community with a too often misogynistic undercurrent, according to several I spoke to. I checked out a few subreddits, and luckily my skin is as thick as rhino's hide after more than a decade of newspaper journalism, because some of what I read was pretty unpleasant, including several threads about people finding pregnant women 'disgusting' and how looking at them makes them 'feel sick'. Sobering reading for someone who was pregnant at the time.

After reading these forums, and then cleansing my palate with several videos of babies and kittens interacting, I can understand why a person without children may not want to be associated with a community that often expresses strong dislike, even hate, for children and their parents. I can understand why communities for those who have difficult feelings about pregnancy (including phobias) need to exist, but some comments were profoundly misogynistic.

After all, we are all part of a collective and a community, and not having your own children doesn't mean that your life is 'childfree', and that the people you love haven't made a different choice to your own. There are many ways to care for children, from being an uncle or godparent to fostering, step-parenting, volunteering or working with them. Perhaps we need to focus less on the act of 'having' a child and more on the act of parenting.

There's also the fact that, for many people, including myself before I became a mother, we are neither 'childless' nor 'childfree', but hover somewhere in between – or oscillate between the two. I have had days where I have spent time with a baby and felt desperately, profoundly childless, only to take to the dancefloor that evening after a dangerous fourth martini and feel blissfully, hedonistically childfree. Perhaps that's one reason why – when absolutely necessary – 'doesn't have children' is the kindest, most neutral descriptor we can hope for. Though we can also hope to be moving away from one's parenting status needing to be defined at all, especially for women, who still face this question far more frequently than men. Language matters, and as ever, it often says more about us and our assumptions than we realise.

The language of maternity is alive and well – so why not expand it to include trans parents?

'Hey, Mama!' This is how I was greeted by a friendly member of staff every morning during my week-long stay in hospital after my baby's birth. Theoretically, I had had my whole pregnancy to get used to the idea of being a mother in the eyes of the world, because almost immediately you become, to the professionals you interact with, 'Mum'. As in: 'could Mum pop herself up on the bed, please?' (Mums seem to do a lot of 'popping'). But nonetheless, it was still surreal to feel my identity shift.

Meanwhile, the baby's father wore a name tag that proclaimed: 'I am [name]. I am husband.' It made me laugh, recalling as it did 'I am woman, hear me roar', or at least a labour ward version of that: 'I am husband, hear me… ask politely once again for pethidine.'

So these were our roles: mother and father, husband and wife. On all the discharge documents, too. Yet if certain media reports are to be believed, one of those terms was under threat: the word 'mother', as a result, apparently, of the push for trans-inclusive language. When, in 2021, Brighton and Sussex maternity services announced they would be adopting gender inclusive language, including terms such as 'birthing parent' and 'chestfeeding', they were accused of misogyny and of 'erasing' womanhood. Though the announcement made clear that the language of women and motherhood would be retained, some reports failed, cynically, to mention this fact, and there was still a social media uproar. (The widespread use of the inclusive term 'birth partner', however, doesn't seem to ever cause such an outcry.)

Fear over the erasure of the language of female biology, especially in maternity services, has become central to the gender-critical discussion of trans versus women's sex-based rights, and yet, as someone who has been pregnant recently, it doesn't seem to bear out. The language of maternity remains heavily gendered: I was almost always mama, mum, mother, a pregnant woman, a lady, a female patient, a breastfeeding mother.

It is true that at times I was a 'pregnant person', though I was never referred to this way by health professionals – it was usually applied by other resources and services, including charities. And in any case, it really didn't bother me. Some aspects of pregnancy can feel dehumanising: I quite liked the fact that I was being given personhood when so often womanhood seems to preclude that.

Yet the notion that trans people want to wipe out the language of maternity persists to the point that it has become, in my view, something of a moral panic.

In her nine years as a midwife, the author Leah Hazard has, to her knowledge, only treated patients that identify as women. However, she feels that inclusive language is an important part of her practice.

'Inclusive language and behaviour aren't about erasing one group. It's about including all groups,' she says. 'It allows all people to feel included and seen and cared for and honoured. And that really is the essence of midwifery.' Instead of seeing inclusive language as a dangerous affront to women, Hazard sees it as part of her duty towards patients. Medical professionals, of course, adapt their language around different patients all the time: they might be working with a mother who has had a double mastectomy after cancer, rendering the language of breastfeeding inappropriate, or whose emergency caesarean means the language of vaginal birth makes her feel terrible.

'If you're in bed one and you want to talk about breastfeeding, I will talk to you about breastfeeding,' says Hazard.

'And if Charlie is in bed two and is a trans man and wants to talk about chestfeeding or body feeding, what skin off my nose, really, is it to talk to Charlie about chestfeeding? None whatsoever... But it just means that I continue to provide that individualised person-centred care that I'm actually duty bound by the regulator to provide.'

The importance of personalised care is even more apparent when I talk to a former colleague and fellow writer Freddy McConnell, a trans man who has just given birth to his second child. 'Throughout both my pregnancies I felt respected and understood by every midwife and doctor I encountered,' he says.

'After my second arrived by emergency C-section, it was incredibly touching and affirming to hear multiple people in the operating theatre spontaneously say, "congratulations, Dad" and "well done, Dad". I didn't have to ask or explain myself. I didn't want special treatment – I just wanted us to be safe and to have a positive birthing experience.' (McConnell notes that the paperwork he was given could have been more inclusive – a point other LGBTQ+ couples have also highlighted.)

I fail to see how anyone could reasonably take umbrage with his words. It seems to be that some of the uproar from the shift towards more inclusive language comes, not as a result of demands from trans people that the word 'mother' be erased, but from organisations and services overcorrecting themselves while seeking to be inclusive.

'I really don't feel comfortable being called a birthing person. I am a mother, I have a baby,' said one NHS source, who complained during a meeting in which replacing 'mother' with 'birthing person' was touted by a colleague. She described the reaction to dealing with this issue as an 'organisational phobia', saying that the focus on this question was overshadowing the more important issue of improving services for everyone. 'I'm not transphobic and I want people to feel comfortable… there needs to be some middle ground.' In the end, her workplace decided on 'women and pregnant people'.

Away from the fury and clamour of social media, professionals are making these decisions every day. They are not always getting it right, but at the heart of their efforts is the desire to create a more inclusive environment for everyone having a baby.

On the day I unexpectedly went into labour, I was re-watching *Seahorse*, a documentary, directed by Jeanie Finlay, about McConnell's journey towards pregnancy and parenthood. All I saw when I watched was another parent, embarking on a new life while negotiating their own specific challenges, as we all do. In this, I felt only solidarity, something we could all do with more of, no matter how we identify.

Millions of men support our abortion rights. We need to help them become stronger allies

As the conversation about abortion rages, it strikes me that I have never heard a man tell his abortion story publicly. The emphasis on disclosure when it comes to abortion means that we have become used to hearing women's stories. But what, if you'll forgive me for ironically borrowing a well-worn phrase, about the men? We hear a lot, too much, from men who are anti-abortion, and little from those who support it, or who have benefited from it.

When the *New York Times* asked men to come forward with their abortion stories, the social media response was mixed. There were the men who thought the whole thing was hilarious, as though the thought of abortion had never troubled them. There were those who thought we shouldn't hear from men about abortion at all, that men should stay out of it. And then there were those who felt perhaps that having men as allies could bolster the cause; that framing it as a 'women's problem' – and not a vital element of family planning that benefits people regardless of gender – plays into the hands of the conservative Christian right.

In the popular cultural imagination of the right, abortion is used by a certain 'type' of woman, an archetypal Jezebel; and even for the left, she's often envisaged as a single, vulnerable young woman. There's an empty space where the man might be. We never see him paying for the abortion and rarely see him attending the clinic; nor do we see him as part of a couple who can't afford to have any more children, or who have made a difficult decision due to a foetal anomaly, or who simply don't want to be parents.

When men are supportive of abortion rights, they often get it wrong, says Joe Strong, a researcher at the London

School of Economics who studies abortion and masculinities. Often, those who support safe and legal abortion mess up by centring themselves, or reinforcing 'patriarchal ideas' by using arguments such as 'hands off my wife's uterus!' or 'I'm doing this for my daughters'. He's noted a trend for articles saying sweeping things like 'abortion is a men's issue too'; but it is not, he says, men's rights that are at stake.

Men should care fundamentally about the reproductive rights of others, whether abortion affects them or not. Of course, in many cases, abortion is the deciding factor in whether a man becomes a father or not, and men will respond emotionally to the life-changing repercussions of this. The crux of the issue, Strong says, is, 'How do we allow men to support women's right to an abortion without elevating their voices over those of women? How do you have a conversation that doesn't imply that a man is a 50 per cent decision-maker in a couple unit when they just aren't?' It's important to hear men's experiences, not only to boost support for women's reproductive rights, but also so that policymaking can reflect reality. It's a delicate balance.

Speak to men privately, and they will be honest about the benefits that abortion has brought to their lives. 'When we found out we were pregnant we were gobsmacked,' one man, Aaron, who was in his early twenties at the time, reflects. He had been dating his girlfriend for a short while and she had been using an IUD. 'When we discussed it, it was clear that we were both on the same page. Neither of us wanted to be parents.'

They had difficulty accessing the procedure after one doctor refused her request, telling her instead to 'pray', meaning she had a later-stage termination than desired.

'Whenever we talked about it afterwards we agreed on it being the right decision – we couldn't have been parents. Both of us have had pretty intense mental health issues since … so

God knows how we could have raised a child together. It was definitely overall a good thing, but a traumatic experience and something that will stay with us both for ever.' They separated but remained friends.

Hearing Aaron's story highlights the role that men can play in the decision not to become a parent: here we see a man who is supportive and sensitive to his partner's feelings, and now, over a decade later, is politically committed to the right to abortion access. Interestingly, Strong's research found that it is not so much a man's opinion on abortion that drives his involvement in decision-making, but 'their feelings on how a pregnancy is going to impact their masculinity'. Often, he says, there's a fear of being seen as a 'deadbeat' dad, a classed, racialised term that carries a lot of stigma. Men ask themselves if a pregnancy will bolster their power in the world (say if they achieve the ideal of father as breadwinner), or not.

'Even though she said she didn't want to keep it, I felt like a piece of shit. I had always been told that it was a man's responsibility to look after any pregnancy they had caused and I felt that I was somehow putting pressure on her … even though she assured me it wasn't the case,' says Aaron, reflecting on the role that ideas of masculinity have played in his own story.

From a policy perspective, Strong argues that we need to grapple with masculinities if we are to truly see a discussion that reflects reality, otherwise many men will continue to link their ability to control another person's body with their conception of manhood. Men's only contribution shouldn't be the reproductive fascism of the Republican Party, or the sort of radicalising 'support groups' we see in the US, where men lament the fatherhood that abortion has 'robbed' them of.

Men who are pro-choice, who have perhaps been told that abortion is a women's issue, may feel the sensitive thing to do is to not speak at all. But can't we find a way for men to talk about abortion without infringing a woman's bodily autonomy, or speaking over her, so that they can become the ultimate allies: men who acknowledge that abortion will never relate to their bodies, but who support it because they believe it is a right.

And, failing that, men can always get their wallets out and donate to feminist organisations. They can use their money, use their patriarchy – as Strong puts it – without needing to use their voices at all.

A dilemma for would-be mothers: date to find the right person – or parent solo?

A few years ago I went for a drink with a female friend who had been dating for some time, but hadn't met anyone in it for the long haul, and she was adamant that she wanted to have children. She felt the ticking of her biological clock acutely, but was frustrated that the men she met acted as though they had all the time in the world. 'I've decided that I'm not going to wait around for some man to get his shit together and commit to me and the possibility of a family,' she announced, citing the Danish phenomenon of the *solomor*, or solo mother. 'I'll give it a couple more years, and then I'm getting a sperm donor and going it alone.'

I admired her. Being single in your thirties is not the quagmire it perhaps was in the 90s, when 'singletons' had to negotiate a world of 'smug marrieds', as Helen Fielding satirised in *Bridget Jones's Diary*. Today's thirty-somethings are more open to alternatives to heterosexual monogamy as a relationship model, being single is less stigmatised, and, in the current post-recession economy, the markers of adulthood are less clear-cut. For the first time, in 2020, the Office for National Statistics found that half of women in England and Wales had not had a baby by their thirtieth birthday, an increase of thirty-two percentage points in fifty years. That is a radical societal shift, and one that reflects women's increasing access to education and career opportunities. But for thirty-something women who want children or are open to the idea, looking for a partner in the modern dating economy can be tricky.

Pippa Bailey is thirty, broke up with her long-term boyfriend a year ago, and is now 'on the apps' in search of a partner. She is one of the female writers who you could say has taken the mantle from Fielding in writing frankly and honestly about the experience of modern romance. In a recent column about the Joachim Trier film *The Worst Person in the World*, whose thirty-something female protagonist is in the midst of an early-thirties crisis, she pinpoints a feeling familiar to many. '[My friends] are buying houses, getting married, having babies, while I continue with "more of the same". I know it is childish and naive, but I find it hard not to feel betrayed, left behind', she wrote.

Bailey thinks she 'probably' wants children, but when she became single, she hadn't anticipated how many people were not looking for a relationship, let alone children. It means the prospect of parenthood requires 'two extra stages of imagining', as she poignantly puts it. She's trying to be more open to the fun of dating without too much pressure, while 'balancing that with wanting to be upfront at the beginning about what you want so that you don't waste your time'.

Apps can facilitate this. Just as you are able to screen partners according to their vaccination status, or whether or not they smoke, you can also filter on the basis of whether someone wants kids or not. Bumble even has a basic info badge where you can state that it's a deal breaker. But Bailey says that a lot of men simply don't answer the question about children.

Men I speak to who are dating tell me that they just don't feel the same fertility pressure as women. 'Twas ever thus, you might say. The sense that women who long for children are a bit 'desperate' is nothing new, but the transactional nature of dating apps casts it into sharp relief.

Though modern women are more confident in expressing all kinds of desires, it strikes me that for a woman to articulate the desire for a child – especially when it feels profound and urgent – remains to some extent taboo.

At least scientific advances mean more women have alternative options. My friend didn't end up needing a donor; she met a lovely man and now has children with him. But I speak to Sioned, thirty-six, who is now heading down that path after splitting from her ex; he already had one child from a previous relationship and didn't want more. After several years of dating, she became increasingly blunt about her desires and found the options for filtering partners helpful, but is less invested in finding someone to embark on parenthood with than she was.

'I like being single, and enjoy dating as a way to connect with new people, but I didn't want my prospects of parenthood to be tied to someone else's shifting desires – especially to a man who doesn't have the same biological time pressures and might change his mind when it's too late for me,' she says. She's inspired by powerful stories of solo motherhood and says queer kinship has taught us there are many kinds of parental models beyond traditional mother–father ones.

As it happens, Sioned has just started dating someone who has said he does want children at some point but, aware the sperm-donor process can take a long time, she has an appointment next week at a clinic. 'I will have to tell him what I'm doing and risk he might not be OK with it, but equally I can't wait around to see if the relationship works and we might try to have a child together.' For women tired of waiting, such conversations – unimaginable centuries ago – look increasingly likely. All power to them for taking action into their own hands.

I see you, single parents. I see your work, your pain – and your joy

Since having my son, I have thought often about single-parent families. 'I don't know how you cope' is a common refrain that you hear from coupled-up parents, but I'm not about to patronise any of you. You cope because you have to, because you love your child or children and they need you. I understand that. I saw my mother do it, and have single parents in my extended family and friendship groups.

What I've been trying to think about is more physical than that. You see, my back hurts. It hurts from lifting the baby, and from walking him up and down every night while singing him maudlin Irish folk songs and, I think, from the fact that as I'm sleeping I unconsciously twist my head towards him, so I can better hear his fluttering breaths. But when my back hurts too much, I pass the baby to my husband, and he starts walking him up and down, and I will go into another room, and sometimes pour a glass of wine.

It's the absence of that small moment of respite that sticks with me. The grinding, physical toll of caring for a child alone, even when it hurts, even when your bones seem to ache.

We don't give single parents much credit. In the UK, the government has actively punished them, penalising them and their children financially in ways both craven and heartless. Reading accounts of how single mothers are struggling in the cost of living crisis brought me to tears last month. It seems to me painfully unfair that, as well as facing all the physical, emotional and financial pressures that come from looking after children alone, single mothers continue to be heavily stigmatised in ways that are both classist and misogynistic, assumed to be 'young, unemployed, feckless, uneducated, hyper-fertile' despite the data showing otherwise.

Then there's the more subtle social exclusion, as couples tend to only socialise with their own. I think (hope?) that my generation is less prone to this particular form of tedious, insecure ostracism, as different lifestyles become more common and many more women especially are actively choosing single motherhood. But the notion of the nuclear family still holds an awful lot of sway.

Sophie Heawood wrote beautifully, in the *Guardian*, about how it feels to live outside that narrative, how she replaced speaking with 'the nod': 'You will do The Nod when the nursery sends your kid home with a Happy Father's Day card that she's been made to copy her name on to. You will employ The Nod when other mums say they know exactly what it's like being a single parent because their lovely husband works abroad for up to two weeks at a time.'

Heawood's memoir, *The Hungover Games*, is a tender and funny account of single parenthood (she calls smug coupled-up parents 'the Hallouminati') in what is becoming a burgeoning genre that is long overdue its time in the sun. It follows Emily Morris's brilliant *My Shitty Twenties*, about the author's experience of an unplanned pregnancy at the age of twenty-two. Séamas O'Reilly's hilarious and heartbreaking *Did Ye Hear Mammy Died?* recounts the experience of being one of eleven siblings raised by a widowed single father.

In poetry, Warsan Shire's work sheds light on the experience of both co-parenting your siblings and raising yourself. Comedy, too, is beginning to reflect and satirise the realities of single parenting, with Katherine Ryan's stand-up and series *The Duchess*, and Diane Morgan's character in *Motherland* acting as important correctives; while Anna Härmälä's cartoons are enlightening and laugh-out-loud funny. But we still need more, and more diverse, depictions.

The relationship between a child and their single parent can be very special, and this is something we rarely see. I have spoken to other adult children of single parents and they often reflect on the intimacy and closeness they feel their childhood has given them. Seeing your parent as a flawed and sometimes vulnerable adult can be its own burden, as can the codependency of such a relationship. But at the same time it can give you a far more nuanced understanding of your parent and their inner emotional life. I have hardly seen this specialness depicted anywhere, I suppose because it kicks so hard against the dominant notion that a child is always better off with two parents at home, and that the children of single parents are deprived by default. To be raised by a lone parent can be a joy and a privilege.

It is true that half of single-parent families live in relative poverty, and this year is going to see more and more single parents struggling to keep their children warm and fed. It is important to highlight that and push for better government support for single parents. But it is also crucial to say to single parents that we see them, we support them and we recognise the work they do every day.

The struggle of fatherhood is real - so why are new dads often invisible in NHS advice?

Before Elliott Rae developed PTSD after the traumatic birth of his daughter, no one had told him that dads could experience birth trauma, too. 'It was a really tough time that included moments of insomnia, anxiety and flashbacks. I became really emotional,' he says. Like many men, he found it difficult to speak about what he was going through. In the years since, he has come to understand the 'societal and cultural norms which contribute to dads feeling pressure to deal with everything by themselves and not talk about the challenges they are going through'.

'I think part of it was imagining an older child, rather than a baby,' another dad, Tom Spencer, tells me, reflecting on his experience of postnatal depression (his daughter is now four). 'There were struggles around breastfeeding. It was really hot that summer. The lack of sleep. Maybe something about the permanence of being a parent? I just felt sad a lot. I remember my partner and me commenting on a day that neither of us cried. I remember putting her in a sling for the first time and being terrified that she had stopped breathing and I'd killed her.'

Dark thoughts began to enter Spencer's mind, followed by guilt. 'I never thought about harming our daughter, but I remember thinking that I might be better able to deal with the grief of her death than the responsibility of keeping her alive and trying to support my partner,' he says.

One in ten men experience anxiety and depression symptoms in the first six months after the birth of a baby, and one in five will experience a mental health problem during pregnancy and the first year after birth. The biggest killer of men under fifty in the UK is suicide – studies have shown that fathers with mental health problems during the perinatal period are up to forty-seven times more likely to be classed as a suicide risk than at any other time in their lives. Yet we hear so little about the impact that pregnancy and birth can have on dads, particularly when they have a history of mental health problems. I've heard women say privately they are concerned about how their partners are coping in the postnatal period, but that the possibility of paternal mental health problems was never mentioned in NCT classes or during engagement with maternity services.

The idea of the strong and silent paternal figure who provides for his family still holds a lot of sway. 'Firstly there was just the shock of responsibility, something I've successfully steered clear of for most of my life,' says Tom Huddleston, a journalist and author who struggled with depression after the birth of his son. 'Secondly, it was just really hard – no one tells you that, or if they do, you don't listen. But as you know, it's just utterly relentless, and the emotional toll is huge. You think – well, this is it now, for 18 years, and however much friends tell you it gets easier, you again don't listen.'

The pressure on men 'to provide unyielding, unidirectional, rock-like support for their partner' is compounded by the feeling that the emotions men are experiencing are not legitimate, according to the sociologists Paul Hodkinson and Ranjana Das, whose book *New Fathers, Mental Health and Digital Communication* is based on interviews with new dads who have experienced mental health problems. These feelings – that their emotions are invalid – mean that they often don't reach out for help until things have reached crisis point. Throughout the pregnancy and birth process they are framed as being peripheral.

According to Adrienne Burgess, the head of research and joint CEO at the Fatherhood Institute, their recent evidence review, 'Bringing Baby Home', revealed a 'dad-shaped hole' in perinatal NHS services. 'They're not being engaged, let alone assessed or referred for support at this crucial time – even though their impacts on mothers' and babies' health and well-being are well-evidenced, significant and wide-ranging, as well as being important in their own right as the child's other parent,' she says. 'We need a paradigm shift in how the NHS thinks about fathers and other non-birthing parents; services should be redesigned to ensure routine, systematic engagement from the first antenatal appointment onwards.'

Peer support is also important. 'I tried talking to a friend about it once, while on a car journey, and he asked me to talk to someone else,' says Tom Spencer, who didn't feel able to confide in his partner or parents. 'I never really asked for help … I like to think I'm not too caught up in trying to be masculine and strong, but once I was in that mind space I didn't feel able to talk about it.'

'Often, male friendships can be surface level, or "shoulder to shoulder",' Rae points out. Men, he says, need face-to-face relationships, especially when their social circles get smaller as they age. 'More social and community groups where men can talk about fatherhood and mental health are really important.'

Huddleston was lucky that his sister is a GP and was able to advise him about postnatal depression in men; his own doctor prescribed him antidepressants, and he gained confidence as a father by taking responsibility for bedtime, which had become a source of anxiety. Spencer shifted his work-life balance and went freelance to spend more time with his daughter.

Rae, meanwhile, set up the platform Music Football Fatherhood for new dads, has edited a book, *DAD: Untold stories of Fatherhood, Love, Mental Health and Masculinity*, and works with NHS trusts to better support fathers during pregnancy and postnatally, as well as running a number of support events.

Partners can play a crucial role, too, in examining their own expectations around fatherhood. 'Just a couple of days ago I was talking to a dad in the gym who said that he is still trying to deal with the trauma of his son's birth five years ago, but his wife and his mum just tell him to get on with it, to stop complaining and be the man of the house,' Rae says. 'We need to challenge and shift our beliefs around what fatherhood is, so we see fathers as caregiving, empathic and nurturing, not just as the stoic breadwinner.'

Having a baby is hard, but the grief of not being able to have one can be even harder

'It's as if you are pressing your nose against the sweet-shop window of life, and you're never ever going to be on the other side.' Jody Day is describing involuntary childlessness. The author and founder of Gateway Women, a global friendship, support and advocacy network for childless women, tells me about what she describes as the 'friendship apocalypse' that can happen between women when one is able to have the children she dreamed of and the other doesn't. After realising that children weren't going to happen for her as a result of 'social infertility' (which means not having children due to circumstance rather than medical issues and is the most common reason for childlessness), Day experienced profound grief. In the process, she lost friends.

'I began to find it incredibly painful to be around my friends with children. And I also realised that I had been the one doing the work to maintain friendships. And when I stopped doing that, when I stopped keeping up with their children's birthdays, with likes on Facebook, with just making sure I was included – what happened? Crickets. It was like I had dropped off the planet. I heard from practically nobody. It was an incredibly lonely period of my life.'

Parenting can be hard, but I've often reflected that it's far, far harder to want a baby and not to have one. This grief is still stigmatised – when Day first started talking about her experience, she was the only one, yet one-fifth of British women will be childless by the time they reach their early forties.

In the course of researching my column, many women got in touch to reflect on how it has impacted their relationships, from both sides of the equation. 'It is difficult feeling outside the club, to perpetually be the group's auntie and uncle, to watch friends announce pregnancies and not feel churned up by resentment and jealousy, ugly emotions I feel guilty for having,' one tells me. Another woman whose friend is going through infertility says: 'It's so hard to know what to say, because I am conscious not to be too positive or negative, as the whole process is highly unpredictable. She is so sad all of the time … Honestly, I don't think I've ever wanted anything as much as she wants this, and it's just heartbreaking to watch.'

The gulf that can emerge during our childbearing years can only deepen with time, as the childless friend slips from the consciousness of the busy parent, or an awkwardness becomes insurmountable, to the point where the two parties are simply performing friendship because they have stopped telling one another the truth. Part of the reason is that envy is such an uncomfortable emotion to admit to. How do you say to someone 'I desperately want what you have' without making them feel uncomfortable? How do you admit feeling angry and resentful at the unfairness of life? 'There's something really cold at the heart of envy that, particularly as women, we don't want to know about. We've been culturally conditioned to be nice,' Day says.

'We're just not raised, as women, to know how to deal with such conflict within our friendships,' says Claire Cohen, author of *BFF? The Truth About Female Friendship*, 'So when it occurs, we end up losing friendships completely. And infertility was one of the areas that seemed to be happening with tragic regularity.' This is why I am trying to be mindful of my friends who don't have children – I don't want to lose them by being one of those tactless parents that Cohen mentions, who says things such as 'At least you can have a lie in!' which amounts, essentially, to a denial of their grief.

And it is grief. Day reminds me that a woman in her thirties who is struggling with involuntary childlessness is only at the beginning of a journey that may mean coming to terms with a different kind of life, from not being involved with the schooling and education system, to not being part of a community of mothers. She will have to grieve not being a grandmother, and may not be treated as a proper adult by her own parents. Talking to Day helps me understand that to not have children when you want them desperately is as profound and transformative as having them, yet this is still rarely recognised despite childless women making up a large part of the population. Day's wisdom is part of the reason that her book *Living the Life Unexpected: How to find hope, meaning and a fulfilling future without children* is recommended by doctors and therapists.

As well as encouraging crucial friendships between childless women to help them in their grief, Day wants to help mothers be better friends to them. This involves recognising that you might not be the best person for them to be around at that time. 'But keep inviting them,' she says. 'If in doubt, never send any baby photos to anyone unless they ask for them. She might say no to coming to birthday parties ... don't presume that they don't want to be part of your life. They just may not be able to cope with it this time, or this week, or this month, or this year.'

Cohen says acknowledging a friend's grief is key, but also notes that infertility is an incredibly difficult thing to be honest about. It remains the fact that parenthood dominates the discourse in a way that a life without much-wanted babies does not. For that to change, parents need to be more comfortable having these difficult conversations, and be less wrapped up in our own lives.

Queer families are teaching us there are many ways to be a mother

What does it mean to be a mother? I've been thinking about that question since before I became one myself, not only in my own writing but while reading the work of others. I've read hundreds of thousands of words on the topic, by writers from a huge range of perspectives and backgrounds, and though it has been hugely rewarding, the question still lingers.

Not long after giving birth, while battling to feed a premature infant with my body, I picked up a copy of Claire Lynch's memoir *Small: On Motherhoods*. It is, among many other things, a tender, powerful reflection on queer motherhood, and on what it means to be a mother when you are not the partner who gives birth to the baby or breastfeeds them, and how it feels to push against those archetypes. It sheds light on how it feels to be embarking on parenthood as an atypical family: the scenes set in pre-natal classes, where Lynch is grouped with the dads, are wryly funny but make a serious point about gender-divided parenting culture. The part where a colleague says: 'Here she comes, the woman who can't even be bothered to give birth to her own children,' (Lynch had had a miscarriage and eventually they decided that her wife would carry the baby) made me gasp.

It has been decades since gay women have been able to start families with the help of fertility treatment, and even longer since they have been doing so without. With some unfair barriers to IVF for lesbian couples having been recently removed, their numbers are only likely to increase. Yet so many of society's ideas about parenthood remain rooted in traditional gender roles. Lynch's use of the plural 'motherhoods' stands in proud contrast to that, a quiet but firm assertion that the idea of a single 'mother figure' needn't be fixed; that it can be up to us how we interpret the role.

Nell Stevens is the author of the novel *Briefly, A Delicious Life* and is pregnant with her second child. Along with her wife, Eley, she is the mother of a toddler, and tells me that, since becoming a parent, she has felt more conflicted about the term 'motherhood'.

'So much [of parenting culture] is "mothers are like this, fathers are like this",' she says. 'With the perceived strengths of motherhood being defined because of the perceived failings of fatherhood. Which is obviously bullshit. I feel very strange about the word motherhood now in ways that I didn't expect to.' The huge identity shift that she was taught to expect when she became a mother didn't happen. 'I wonder if a lot of that is because, in straight relationships, the differences between the partners become so stark, and that in turn shapes your idea of yourself in a shocking way.'

I agree. I think in heterosexual relationships, no matter how egalitarian you try to be, societal gender roles intervene. When there are two mothers, perhaps there is more freedom to design your own roles. That's not to say that there aren't still differences between the birthing parent and the non-birthing parent, which can make the shift challenging in all sorts of ways, but, as Stevens says: 'it has freed us up to parent more authentically, I think, rather than going "I'm the dad, therefore I do this".'

As is often the case, it's the surrounding culture that has posed challenges, from midwives assuming Eley was Nell's mum ('She's younger than me!' says Nell) to romantic ideas of fatherhood and dads being the ones who fix everything. 'Parenthood is the only space in which I've been made to feel really weird,' she says. 'It's still a little bit shocking to a surprising amount of people.'

Speaking with the journalist Sian Norris, who grew up in a gay household of two women (her mum was in a straight marriage with her dad, then met her female partner when Sian was a young child), there's a sense that society has moved on from the days of section 28 and Aids prejudice – but not as much as we could have done. 'I wasn't open about growing up in a gay household until my late teens, really, because anything "gay" was seen as bad or disgusting or sick when we were younger,' she says. 'We were warned that we would be raised as "freaks" and that we would turn out to be drug addicts or child abusers ... this was the common narrative of that time.' The fact that there was no 'male influence' in the household was something people couldn't get their heads around.

'I felt a lot of anger about section 28 making my family "fake" and unspeakable,' she tells me. 'And I still experienced homophobia from work colleagues in recent years, which was a shock after being open about it for so long.' That pernicious phrase that 'a child needs a mother and a father' persists to this day. According to a 2020 study, one in three lesbian mothers in Britain has experienced homophobia from other parents, while the same proportion have children who have been bullied for having two mums.

Which is why it's so radical and beautiful that we are seeing so much writing about queer motherhood, from Bernardine Evaristo's Booker-winning *Girl, Woman, Other* to an upcoming memoir by Kirsty Logan, *The Unfamiliar*, to Lynch's *Small*. The beauty of the latter is its quiet assertion that what makes a mother is not biology but presence, those tender moments of care, the hard graft, the exhaustion, the fear: sharing and steering that child's journey of wonder and discovery as they grow.

Many people celebrate friends' pregnancies – with no way of expressing their own longing for children

I tried to look up baby fever, but all that came up is information about an infant's vitals and how to take their temperature. It's more of an American term, baby fever. In British English, we are more likely to say broody, which comes from hens, but there's something benign and cosy-sounding about that word. A friend once asked me if I was clucking, to mean 'do you feel a desire to get pregnant?' I had never heard it before, but again, it was too nice for what I was feeling, which was at times dark and desperate and jealous and mean.

In my memoir, *The Year of the Cat*, published in 2023, I try to pinpoint that feeling of longing, because it seemed to me that literature had still not fully explored it, perhaps because it can feel so deep and primal and beyond words. In the end, I am forced to resort to Welsh to describe it. I use the word *hiraeth*, which means to feel longing for a place or a person or a time that feels like home but may never have existed except in your imagination.

That's as close a description as I have been able to reach, and I think it goes some way to explaining that feeling of recognition that people describe when they meet their child for the first time, an 'oh, it's you'. Laura Marling's song 'For You', is one of the few tracks I can think of that put these emotions into words. That song is now on the baby's playlist, and every time I listen to it, I think about the longing.

Of course, I have been lucky, because my wish came true. Perhaps that is why I am able to write about it now, though as I was writing my book I was not pregnant, so there was always a risk that it would be published and I'd be asked about these difficult emotions without them being resolved. Regardless of what happened in my own story, though, I wanted to write it for all the women – and men, because men can feel a strong longing for a child too – who are sitting with these often unspoken feelings who raise glasses of champagne to their friends' happy announcements but cry on the way home and then feel guilty, because that knot of feeling is primal and complicated and sometimes ugly. It can be hard to say to people you love that you want what they have. Sometimes it's easier to just leave the WhatsApp group or skive the baby shower.

When I did some research about the longing – of which, as with so many things to do with female reproduction, there is of course little written – most papers and studies suggested that the visceral physical and emotional feeling of wanting to have a baby is largely socialised as opposed to hormonal. A 2011 Kansas State University study named three factors: having positive interactions with babies, such as playing and cuddling; the extent of negative exposure to babies, which dampens the desire; and how someone views the 'trade-offs' of parenthood. 'Those with baby fever see only the positive impacts on their life,' a fertility expert said in one article about baby fever.

Far be it for me to argue with experts, but I know what I felt. I was acutely aware of the negative impact that having a baby could have on my life, and was for a long time in a sort of paralysis. But it didn't change the visceral longing I felt, or which many others describe. Anecdotally, friends have said that their longing ebbs and flows with their cycles. Older women who felt it pre-menopause have also said that it wanes with time (though others have had to learn to live with it their entire lives). Some women, and again, men, have never felt it at all, and I've always wondered if there are evolutionary reasons for this, because to have every member of a tribe occupied with childcare is hardly going to help when trying to ward off predators. Are the women I know who have never wanted children simply immune to social pressure? Or is it something inherent? Perhaps we are all just socialised to blame our hormones. Whatever the reason, they are sick of being told that their feelings will change.

All I know is that, until we speak honestly about longing, at least within our families and friendship groups, it will continue to come out in ways that can be uncomfortable. When a friend said that her sister had ruined every single family occasion for this reason, I could see both sides. Fertility message boards and support groups can offer some comfort to those going through the longing, but for many childless couples it remains a difficult thing to speak about. This is one of the few things in life that our capitalist economy cannot provide a failsafe solution for. You can try to spend your way out of the problem, but there are no guarantees. The whims of the female body remain mysterious and ungovernable. That's why the longing is still so stigmatised. To want what you perhaps can't have, the desperation of that feeling, it's something many would rather not know about. Which is why I felt compelled to write about it.

Having a baby after pregnancy loss is a joy. But it may never wipe the slate clean

'It's the idea that everything is healed.' Jennie Agg is talking to me about miscarriage. Or, specifically, how it feels to have a baby after miscarriage – or miscarriages, plural; Agg had four before she gave birth to her boy. *Life, Almost* – her book detailing her experiences and investigating why miscarriage still remains such an under-researched and under-acknowledged experience – is a vital examination of the subject, with each chapter given the title of some of the false, trite or dismissive things people say: 'It's just nature's way', 'it's not a real baby yet', 'everything happens for a reason'.

In a book full of insights, perhaps one of the most affecting is the dawning understanding of the legacy that pregnancy loss can have. There is still an absurdly prevalent notion that finally getting a healthy baby – as most couples who experience miscarriage will – somehow wipes the slate clean, and makes everything that has happened in the past melt away. 'Any residual grief, trauma or yearning is supposed to be washed away by the arrival of a longed-for child,' she writes. 'After all – you got what you wanted, didn't you?'

Agg admits that she herself, who had been just so desperate to get to a point where she could bring a baby home, even believed this to an extent. She notes that most miscarriages we hear about in the media are stories told in retrospect, from the perspective of a safe place of 'success'. ('We do not see miscarriage lived, only reported,' is one of the many standout lines from the book.) And so they are treated as blips in a journey that are now in the past, rather than experiences that might continue to reverberate in the present. While women might feel more comfortable talking about miscarriage from the perspective of now being a mother – and others, I suspect, may feel relieved from some of the discomfort and awkwardness they feel when it's talked about – Agg argues that this framing means that we do not see a fully nuanced picture of miscarriage. Nor do those with a history of miscarriage always feel able to talk about parenting and parenthood in all its complexity.

Because how, for instance, do you say that you're not enjoying it, that you're finding it difficult, when you wanted it so desperately? Agg writes that she often opted to stay silent, not only about the challenges of motherhood, but also about the positives, aware of how they could wound those who are going through miscarriage. The way other people behave towards you changes too, she notes. 'I think people no longer feel that awkwardness or that pressure or that discomfort ... very quickly, they proceed to treat you like any other person.' And so she found herself being asked, glibly, 'Do you think that you'll have another?' even though the reasons for her repeated losses were never discovered or resolved.

She tells me how miscarriage meant that for the first six months of her baby's life, every moment just felt incredibly precious, that she felt determined not to take everything for granted. But with that comes 'an awareness of how easily it might not have happened, how fragile it is', and a sadness at what they had been missing for so long. She acknowledges, too, an anxious hypervigilance in how she parents, though she tries to steer clear of the language of trauma. Many parents worry about developmental milestones, of course, or will feel on edge when their baby has a bad wheezy cough, but a history of miscarriage can exacerbate anxiety further.

One in five women who experience early miscarriage are afflicted with PTSD-like symptoms, and we know that it is a predictor of postnatal depression and/or anxiety. Despite this, healthcare professionals doing postnatal checks are still not advised to treat pregnancy loss as a contributing factor, or to ask about it. Even in the medical profession, it seems, miscarriage can be treated as irrelevant once a woman has 'successfully' given birth.

Agg says that it would have made such a difference if it had been raised, or if it had been acknowledged that it's not only normal to find parenthood hard, but that such a medical history might make it more so. Instead, you can end up with a romanticised ideal of what parenthood is going to be like, while also being completely unprepared for it, because you don't want to tempt fate by organising anything or doing too much research.

Of course, how a person parents after miscarriage not only affects them and their partner, but also the child that has been born. Agg is resolute that she doesn't want to treat her son like a 'miracle baby', or burden him with too much meaning, so that he grows up 'in the shadow of putative children'. At the end of the book, she writes of how a friend told her that in her religion the souls of babies lost in pregnancy are believed to be reincarnated in in subsequent children. It is not an idea that everyone might find comforting, though Agg does. More interesting though, I think, is her discovery that embryos shed cells into a mother's bloodstream that can remain in her blood and tissue for years afterwards. So, yes, as a result of this microchimerism, microscopic traces of one baby could go on to exist in another.

But what strikes me even more is how this process is, in its way, a perfect metaphor for grief and its residues; how the things that happen to our bodies never truly leave us. Particularly the visceral grief that can come from the loss of the much-wanted pregnancy that might leave traces for even decades afterwards. We should recognise and honour that pain, and support those enduring it.

George Eustice's drivel about stay-at-home mums reinforces the trap set by society for women

Since becoming a mother, I've found myself thinking a lot about stay-at-home mums.

What a job. It is hard graft – round-the-clock physical, mental and emotional labour. Stay-at-home parenting is mostly undertaken by women, but does that mean that it's our 'natural nurturing role', as the Tory MP George Eustice said? He argues that the government is prioritising childcare policy at the expense of incentivising women to stay at home. 'Fathers, of course, have a very strong paternal desire to spend time with their children, but you can't get away from the way we are biologically wired – and the maternal instinct is a strong one,' he said. 'It is generally the case that mothers in particular will want, if they can, to spend that time with their young children.'

Many of us would disagree with the idea that women are biologically programmed to perform all of the work of stay-at-home parenting, or that men don't want to be central to their children's lives. It feels terribly convenient, doesn't it?

Yet our ideas of fatherhood are shifting. Both the Fatherhood Institute and Dr Anna Machin, one of the UK's leading evolutionary anthropologists and author of *The Life of Dad*, have deplored the comments for the outdated, ignorant and insulting drivel they are. Machin in particular pointed out how unsupported men are when they want to be present parents in their children's lives.

Not all dads. Some use 'weaponised incompetence' when it comes to childcare. Often both halves of a heterosexual couple will engage in the delusion that the father is useless, so the mother has to do everything. The woman, therefore, becomes 'the expert in the baby'. And so she never lets him learn, or he never bothers, and he never becomes the dad he could be.

Why do I mention this? Because, in this way, society has been performing a sort of weaponised incompetence when it comes to childcare policy for decades now: 'it's easier if you do it.' Society hasn't been supporting women to stay at home, but it has been expecting it.

It isn't easier. Women often feel they have no choice. Hence the need for affordable childcare. Of course, if a woman chooses to be a stay-at-home mother, then that choice should be supported. Some women can't wait to get back to the office, but some are heartbroken to be putting their babies in full-time nursery and would rather stay home, but can't.

Stay-at-home mums are often left out of these discussions because their existence is inconvenient to both sides. Women who actively want to be stay-at-home mums are uncomfortable for some feminists to contemplate because they have traditionally been so lionised.

And the stay-at-home mum is threatening to the other side of the debate because capitalism relies on free domestic labour. She can be encouraged and deified as long as she doesn't consider what she is doing as work worthy of financial recompense. The minute she does that, she becomes dangerous.

What is Eustice suggesting we do about stay-at-home mums, I wonder? Because if he believes that we should be like Finland, where the government subsidises parents who would prefer to care for their young children at home, then we are probably in agreement. That all may sound a bit too modern to his ears: after all, it includes dads. Though the policy has been criticised as one designed to keep women at home, really what it offers is choice.

Another aspect is class. Stay-at-home mums are considered desirable as long as they are not a 'drain' on society. The ideal of the stay-at-home mum is rooted in middle-class values – supported by her husband, aesthetically pleasing, smiling and functional. Never angry or poor or mentally unwell.

I say this as a woman who was raised by a middle-class, stay-at-home mother on benefits, who is a feminist, who made her daughter a feminist, one grateful that her mother was there each day when she came home from school, who could never be a stay-at-home mother herself without going mad, but who has opted to work part-time so she can care for her son. Complicated, but not unfathomable. None of this is, as long as we all value the work that women do and support their choices.

'One and done' parents are some of the most thoughtful and compassionate I have met

'Aren't you worried they'll be lonely?' This is the question that the parents of only children are probably asked the most, and the one that is mentioned again and again when I asked for 'one and done' parents to get in touch. Although 'one and done' parenting is on the rise, and in some countries only children are becoming the norm, the stigma against single-child families is real. Stereotypes about only children being spoilt, obnoxious or lonely persist.

What my callout on social media revealed is that there are many persuasive economic and social reasons for deciding to only have one child, and though they can be as diverse and complex as families themselves, there are some common threads.

The financial cost of being a parent in Britain – the astronomical cost of childcare, not being able to afford a larger home – was a major theme, as was the impact that motherhood continues to have on women's careers. The climate emergency was another. One mother, who asked to be anonymous because it upsets her own mother so much when she says that she won't have any more children, wrote how 'the backdrop to my first trimester was two 35+ degree heatwaves. I'm terrified for my boy's future'.

Another frequent theme was the lack of support, and a palpable sense that the UK is particularly unwelcoming for parents. 'There is no "village",' wrote one mother, whom I'll call Angie. The fact that she had a baby later in life means that her parents are elderly and her siblings have their own families. She found the early stages of motherhood 'extremely difficult', suffering from postpartum anxiety, and decided not to risk her mental health again, with the impact that could have on her happy son. Angie is far from the only parent who contacted me citing mental health as a contributing factor to her decision-making. Traumatic experiences during birth were a common reason – the makers of the podcast *Only You* highlight the role of pregnancy complications that are likely to recur.

'I feel like the experience very nearly broke me and the thought of doing that all again with a toddler is enough to trigger an anxiety spike …' wrote another mother, Rosie. 'I truly feel like I barely survived the first time round and I have no desire to put myself in the same space again.'

The belief that 'one and done' parents are being selfish in not giving their offspring a sibling is widespread, but in speaking to parents, I actually found the opposite: they put the happiness and welfare of their existing child front and centre, whether it is deciding that a new sibling means they would not be able to devote enough time or resources to their first child, or that risking their mental health is in no one's best interests. I was moved by the compassion and the thoughtfulness with which 'one and done' parents approached the issue.

It is a shame that many can't see the decision to have an only child for what it often is: an act of responsible parenting. For Lauren Sandler, the author of *One and Only: The Freedom of Having an Only Child, and The Joy of Being One*, an answer lies in our changing social structures. 'Larger families made sense when we worked the land, when we had high infant mortality rates,' she says. 'Your family was your labour force, your insurance policy, your tribe. Since that time, especially since women have needed to make a living, and, beyond that, have chosen to have careers … a lasting bias strikes me as serving the old structure: women doing unpaid labour at home. The more kids, the more labour. And the more labour the less active citizenship, the less freedom for spending hours as we please.'

Being 'one and done' is certainly more common, so is it good or bad being an only child?

It is interesting to me that the parents of only children are frequently challenged about the potential negative impact on their offspring, but we never really speak about what being a part of a large family can mean for a child's emotional well-being. 'I was never jealous of my friends' sibling setups: it seemed either an annoying younger sibling was always trying to join in, or that an older sibling was exasperated by our unwanted attention. Their houses seemed noisy and chaotic, with someone inevitably in tears or screaming,' wrote one only child. As Sandler notes, decades of studies show that only children fare just as well, or better, even, than kids with siblings, and their parents tend to be happier, too, with lives that ideally offer more freedom, pleasure and fulfilment.

While those who want more children but feel grief and anger at being robbed of the choice by circumstance deserve support, it must also be recognised that being one and done can be joyful and positive. The way forward is, I think, to highlight these pluses of being and having an only child.

Notably, the parents who seemed most at ease with their decision to have only one had been happy only children themselves. 'I had a wonderful upbringing with no siblings; I have a great relationship with my parents and was always treated as an equal, and got their undivided attention,' says Rosie. 'I love having the physical, emotional and financial capacity to give my daughter everything she needs, while maintaining my own identity and independence – something I fear I might lose if I had another child.'

Emotions around infertility can be raw. Let's talk about them with solidarity

I first came across the idea of 'fertility privilege' in a podcast by the author Elizabeth Day, who has been admirably open about her desperate desire to be a mother after repeat miscarriages and fertility treatment. The podcast made me cry, though Day would be well within her rights to tell me to stuff my tears, because I got my baby. I joined the club. I have what she terms 'fertility privilege', i.e., I have conceived and carried a child without too much difficulty.

In an article that caused something of a furore, Day wrote: 'We rightly talk about privilege in this era of social change – an era marked by Black Lives Matter and #MeToo – but hardly anyone acknowledges fertility privilege. Those of us who have had complicated journeys to parenthood are only too aware of its existence … I know how it feels to be the infertile one in a world of apparent abundance. I wouldn't post about my glorious babies on social media in much the same way as I wouldn't post about my expansive mansion or my fleet of Bentleys (not that I have any of those), because it's thoughtless to those who don't have these things.'

There can be a certain self-satisfaction to motherhood, as reflected in the photographs we post and the things we say to each other when childless women aren't present (not to mention the thoughtless things we can say when they are). Many mothers are mindful of their good fortune that their children are here and – by the grace of God – safe and well. There is a feeling of relief, of being smiled on by biology. There is, of course, the boundless love which can seem all-consuming and can manifest as exclusivity.

Those living with infertility seem to more commonly embrace the concept of fertility privilege, or feel acknowledged by it; the author Jennie Agg has written movingly on the complacency she encountered around pregnancy as she endured repeat miscarriages. Many women with children also expressed admiration for the term as a way of vocalising how lucky they felt to easily conceive.

More, though, found it a divisive term or felt it lacked nuance. Many mothers have also experienced miscarriage and fertility issues. Fertility privilege arguably flattens the experience of pregnancy and childbirth, which can be fraught with difficulty. One woman who has struggled with infertility writes to me that the comparison with material luxuries is inappropriate – after all, children aren't commodities and most people have them. She compares all the #blessed posts on social media to sharing pictures of abundant food when we know others live with food insecurity.

Mothers already feel as though they aren't granted the space they need to speak openly: that they must tiptoe around. 'It seems like sometimes we need to apologise for being mothers and aren't allowed space to talk honestly about the ups and downs without sugarcoating it so much it becomes meaningless,' one told me. 'Talk of privilege feels so inappropriate and lacking in empathy,' says another, who is struggling after a traumatic birth. 'Mothers simply cannot condemn themselves to any more guilt than we are already socially conditioned to endure. We are maxed out,' says another.

I struggle with the idea that whether an egg becomes fertilised or not – a lottery – should carry moral implications. Fertility is not structural or fixed – it changes month by month or year by year. 'Fertility can be the opposite of desirable for a lot of people – who really don't want to get pregnant. It can be a burden or a threat to them,' writes one woman, who says she had periods of 'hyperfertility' that resulted in two abortions.

Another highlights victims of rape who become pregnant. 'Being fertile doesn't mean the end of the story,' says a mother who had two healthy children but was then diagnosed with cancer.

Furthermore, talk of fertility privilege is in itself synonymous with a certain background; these are often middle-class women usually talking about other middle-class women. That is not to deny their pain, but to be fertile and working class, on benefits or a teenager, is not culturally prized in the same way. It is actively condemned. Pregnancy and childbirth often lead to discrimination and marginalisation.

Still, I admire Day's attempts to widen the language around miscarriage, infertility and not-motherhood. To quote the poet Sandeep Parmar: 'Taxonomies of grief elude the non-mother, the unmothered, the-anything-but-this-fact.' There is so much hidden pain, apparent to anyone who has looked at fertility forums.

As one reader reflected, getting pregnant after a year and a successful course of treatment would be considered 'privileged' to others. Some forum users who have never become pregnant will intimate that even a woman undergoing the trauma of repeat miscarriage is somehow 'lucky', because she can 'at least get pregnant'. Many of these emotions are raw and ugly, which is why people shy away from discussing them face to face. Day's radical honesty opens up the conversation.

There is so much more at play, though, when it comes to having children, than mere biology. 'I'm not sure that I feel as privileged in my fertility as I do in the complicated intertwining of privileges which allowed me to have them (being in a heterosexual relationship, finding someone who agreed to have children earlier than they planned, the financial stability to do so, a strong familial support network),' says a woman who had children young because of endometriosis. I do wonder where it all ends: do those with female bodies have fertility privilege above gay men? What about those who can afford fertility treatment, even if it is ultimately unsuccessful?

And what of single women? Reading Amy Key's *Arrangements in Blue*, a beautiful memoir about a life lived without romantic love, I am moved by her descriptions of longing for a child, her lack of bitterness and generosity to those in her life who have what she so craved. That is not to say that to be bitter is inappropriate – too often women are told to mask these difficult emotions. More that Key seems less interested in the privileges that divide us than in the forms of love that can unite us, whatever they may be, and expand our understanding of what it means to have a life well lived, fostering solidarity between all women, whatever our journeys.

No woman should have to give birth alone. Pregnant asylum seekers need our support

It feels trite to say that pregnancy and birth can be the most vulnerable experiences in a woman's life, and yet there is a need to say it, still, because so much of that physical experience feels untranslatable. There was certainly a moment while I was giving birth when I felt acutely that my future sanity was in jeopardy. What saved me was my husband, my birth partner.

The role of the birth partner has increased in importance in recent decades; we are far removed from the days when our grandfathers were told to stay outside the birthing room because of the old belief that men would faint. Women being forced to give birth alone during the pandemic has rightly been a source of outrage, and yet this is the situation facing some single women every day. This is especially true of migrant women, who lack the support network so many of us are lucky to have. Yet I have rarely heard anyone express concern about the lonely births that asylum seekers often endure.

A birth partner serves many functions – they ask for water, pain relief, examinations when you can't. They seek clarification from medical professionals about what is happening. They stroke your back and absorb your fears and your fury. Migrant women are especially vulnerable and disadvantaged, because they do not know the healthcare system, may not speak the language, and often have no family support. Many will have a history of trauma, compounded by negotiating what is an increasingly hostile environment. To give birth alone in this context is a daunting prospect indeed.

It is in response to this set of circumstances that Amma Birth Companions, a Glasgow charity, was founded. The project trains volunteers to support women who would otherwise give birth alone. Since it was founded in 2019, it has supported almost 300 women, most of whom are in the asylum process and at least a third of whom are survivors of trafficking. Language, cultural barriers and poverty are factors in their lack of access to services, and they need help navigating the system. Pregnancy and childbirth can interact with pre-existing mental health conditions such as PTSD to cause perinatal mental health problems, so such support is vital.

The project is flourishing, and has now expanded beyond its original remit, offering postnatal support, antenatal education and advocacy. It's an inspiring example of women supporting women in the community, recognising that it is inhumane for any woman to give birth alone. When it comes to childbirth, this is what solidarity looks like.

There is no one type of volunteer: there are mothers, grandmothers, students and those who don't want to have children. Once a pregnant woman has been matched with one of their pool of sixty volunteers, ideally one who speaks the same language, that volunteer might visit her at home two or three times during the third trimester, assisting with planning for the birth, packing a hospital bag, signposting to other services, and providing antenatal education, as well as crucial emotional and moral support.

Then, from thirty-seven weeks, the birth companion is on call to attend the birth. To know there is someone waiting, only a phone call away, to be your advocate must be a weight off any expectant mother's mind, but especially so in a strange, often hostile country. We all need someone to hold our hand at times like these.

Comfort was one of the first women to be supported by Amma when she delivered her son Simon by planned caesarean section three years ago. At the time, she had serious mental health problems and support had fallen away due to the pandemic. 'Just to have somebody there was good, as I was really worried about how it was just me. It was really scary. They stayed by me, stood by me, spoke to the midwife and the doctor on my behalf. They were more like family,' she told me.

She hadn't intended to breastfeed but with support she decided to do it and ended up loving the experience, breastfeeding Simon for eighteen months. It goes to show how the work of birthing partners can help to shape a mother and child's lives. Comfort was so moved by the support she received she is now an active volunteer and a member of the board, advocating for other women.

Amma is not the only organisation offering birth companionship – they exist elsewhere, from Project Mama in Bristol to London's Happy Baby Community. With the passing of the illegal migration bill, pressure on these organisations is likely to increase as they try to fill the gaps in support provision. Women fleeing persecution who arrive in the UK via 'irregular' means will be prevented from claiming asylum and detained indefinitely, with no exemption for those who are pregnant, removing the vital protection introduced in 2016 by the seventy-two hour time limit on the detention of pregnant women.

This will only increase the barriers these women face, from not accessing services for fear of deportation to the life-threatening implications of being placed in detention. The 72-hour detention time limit for pregnant women has been maintained, but many more women still need support and companionship during pregnancy and childbirth. To choose to give that, as Comfort and her fellow volunteers are doing, is a powerful gift indeed.

We all want better for our children than we had – but Britain's housing crisis is crushing that dream

Before we decided to have a baby, I thought a lot about what being a mother would be like, but there were some respects in which my imagination failed me. Both are related to my living environment. I live in a first-floor flat with quite a few steps leading up to the front door from street level, and it did not occur to me that this would be what might politely be termed a 'complete and utter ball-ache', both in respect of getting myself and the baby outside, but also his many effects, meaning it requires at least two trips and, unless I am using the Babyzen Yoyo, which is extremely light, the assistance of my husband or sometimes my very kind neighbour. Without that pram and someone there to assist, I'd basically be housebound, which makes me feel pathetic and a tad vulnerable. (For a while I could pop the baby on a blanket in the communal hall while lugging the pram down the steps, but now that he is mobile he's on a kamikaze mission to go headfirst after me.)

The other was toys. For some reason, I had not realised that there would be so many toys, and that not tripping over those toys in the dark at 3.55 a.m. when retrieving a bottle would become quite key.

So when a friend falls pregnant now, I tend to gently highlight these two things, especially the former, so that she can be prepared. Although what tends to happen is that her housing situation comes with its own issues, as in the case of the friend who moved to a ground-floor apartment in preparation, but has found the neighbourhood outside it to feel crime-ridden and lacking in green space. Having a baby changes your approach to housing, both in a practical and an emotional sense. The way you use space changes, as does the way that you feel within that space. It's all for someone else, now, and so your home's shortcomings feel more depressing and distressing than ever.

I write this as a renter in an area that has gentrified so completely in the past decade that any former resident who comes to see you spends at least the first ten minutes swearing in disbelief. As such, it's been a lovely place in which to have a baby, and there is still a feeling of community here. On the other hand, it can be quite fatiguing being surrounded by millionaires, and now that I'm a parent, the absurdity of the wealth divide in my borough hits even harder. That there should be babies in beautifully appointed nurseries in Victorian townhouses, all decorated in various shades of sad beige (the satirical term used to describe the way upper-middle class parents eschew colour in pursuit of a Scandi aesthetic), a stone's throw from children living in appalling cramped conditions: it breaks my heart.

It's not that I begrudge the friends and acquaintances who have made it onto the property ladder (most of them), usually with huge cash injections from family. They are admirably candid about this. But living side by side with them at times makes that lifestyle feel achievable, when in fact you might as well wish that you had won the lottery. So successful has been the media manipulation around the housing crisis that to be renting at my age and stage of life feels like a personal failure, even though I know objectively that it isn't. At one point a few years ago buying a house somewhere else in the UK started to look possibly achievable, though relocation work-wise would have been a challenge, and then Liz Truss happened.

There are many thousands of others in the same boat, or worse off, and many thousands of others living with mortgage terror, working multiple jobs in fear of losing their homes. The social contract in terms of being able to provide an affordable, comfortable home for your family by working hard has completely broken down. The landlord class continues to leech off the younger and the poorer. I think about the parents who are waiting to have the lift repaired for the seventh time, the ones who already have too many children in too little space, or who have decided that they can't have another despite desperately wanting one because there's nowhere to put them.

I think a lot about Awaab Ishak, the two-year-old boy who died because of a respiratory condition caused by exposure to mould at his Rochdale home. Especially last winter, when the black mould bloomed on our own windowsills, and while my husband scrubbed and scrubbed, I sobbed and sobbed because our son had needed help to breathe when he was born early, and I was scared for his tiny lungs. I couldn't write about it at the time. I felt ashamed. Because how could someone with all my privileges, someone writing a parenting column for a national newspaper, be in such a situation?

I consider myself lucky. I have a landlord, Clarion Housing, that will eventually replace the windows, though it took two years for them to fix the crumbling brickwork that made my son's room so damp, and they are yet to make the collapsing wall in the back garden safe, or provide an outside tap for a paddling pool, or fix the hob in the kitchen. But it's better than what most tenants get (the bar is very low).

If you're reading this in your beautiful, secure home, you are one of the fortunate ones – there are millions of parents out there who are not. I suppose I want them to feel seen. Because it used to be taken for granted that you could give your children a better life than you yourself had, and in the past decade we've lost that principle. I don't know how we find it again.

In the rage over the two-child benefits cap, one fact gets lost: this is state control of women's bodies

Since becoming a parent, I no longer have much time. There are 4,524 unread emails in my inbox, and I only recently got a pedicure despite the fact that it's been at least thirteen months since I've been able to see my feet again. But it turns out that I do have time to be properly livid with the Labour Party, which is refusing to budge on its failure to promise to scrap the two-child benefits policy, despite the fact that it has pushed a quarter of a million children into poverty and 850,000 even deeper below the breadline.

Perhaps it's tone deaf to talk of pedicures in the same breath as child poverty, but these small things mothers do for themselves – getting our roots done, or even just a long, hot bath – help us stay sane. The toll that parenting takes on your body doesn't stop after birth: it is physical, bone-aching work, and birth of course can lead to myriad long-term health issues. These small acts of self-care matter; they make us feel worth something.

They are also the first things to go in times of financial hardship. We all make sacrifices for our children's well-being to different extents, and in a cost of living crisis money for such things might be needed elsewhere. Pedicures are the least of it: there will be many women going hungry in this country today so that their children can eat.

The effects of the two-child policy, which limits benefits to the first two children born into a family, have been widely and rightly condemned. The bitter internal row in the Labour Party over this especially cruel and nasty legislation shows what an emotive issue it is.

It goes without saying that punishing innocent children for their parents' apparent reproductive profligacy is a heinous political strategy. And for what? It hasn't even worked. The social policy professor Jonathan Bradshaw has called it 'morally odious' and worse than the 1834 legislation that brought workhouses into existence. Considering how that policy broke up families, starved children and essentially warehoused 'undesirables' in a way the Nazis would later replicate, that is quite a strong statement.

But what is less discussed, and which I can't stop thinking about, is its impact on the female body. Philip Alston, the UN's then special rapporteur on extreme poverty and human rights, said that the UK's benefits system was so sexist that it might as well have been conceived by 'a group of misogynists in a room' determined to make a system that works for men and not women. There was, rightly, outrage about the 'rape clause' in this policy that requires that women who have had a third child as a result of rape prove it to the government in order to claim for benefits, but less about the fact that the reproductive rights of every single woman in the UK have been quietly encroached upon.

Essentially what we have here is the legislating of the female body, in plain sight, yet with none of the outrage and fury that we see over abortion rights. In forcing women to choose between abortion and poverty, the policy appears specifically designed to limit women's reproductive choices. But because, I suspect, societal ideas about working-class maternal fecklessness are so ingrained, even people who consider themselves socially progressive might um and ah when asked their views on women on benefits reproducing.

And so there are no marches. Two years ago, two single mothers and their children valiantly challenged the legislation in court on the basis that it was discriminatory, but they lost. (It was noted in the coverage that one of the mothers had become pregnant despite being on the pill and that the other was in low-paid work: i.e., they were the 'right sort' of single mothers). In the judgement the supreme court president, Lord Reed, said that while the policy had a disproportionate impact on women, Parliament had decided that was outweighed by the importance of its economic aims. How chilling I find that sentence. How chilling we should all find it.

But as my own (single) mother frequently says: ''Twas ever thus'. Our bodies are under the bus, again, and scarcely anyone seems to care. They are, I suppose, the wrong sorts of bodies: poor bodies, Black and Brown bodies (the policy disproportionally affects women of colour), disabled bodies. Even if your body is none of these things, and you're one of the women getting monthly pedicures, it is a dangerous precedent that has been set; and in the spirit of maternal – nay, female – solidarity, we should all abhor it.

As Sian Norris, the author of *Bodies Under Siege*, tells me: 'The two-child policy seeks to legislate over women's bodies, treating women's wombs as something that can and should be arbitrated on by the state. It ties into ideas of women's wombs being public property, which in turn links to anti-abortion ideology – ironic considering the policy is pushing some women to terminate wanted pregnancies as they can't afford to care for a third or fourth child.'

She added: 'There is a specific class-based element to this that states that if you are on a low income, then you are not entitled to make your own decisions about pregnancy, fertility and your family.'

A Labour Party without the moral courage to challenge this policy is unworthy of the name. Set against the background of demographic panic about the birth rate, its stance is even more nonsensical. The birth rate is plummeting, and women are ending wanted pregnancies.

In 2020 the British Pregnancy Advisory Service noted that since the policy was introduced, the proportion of abortions to women with two or more children had risen by 16.4 per cent. They're the wrong sort of women to be having babies, though. We don't want migrant or impoverished mothers, and we don't want their children, who, if they have the audacity to exist, must be punished. We want only the right sort. 'Twas ever thus.

Formula milk advert restrictions are patronising – let parents decide what's best

Like many parents, I wasn't aware of the laws around the promotion of baby formula until I needed to buy it, to feed my pre-term, extremely hungry baby. I discussed the stigma with a friend who was also formula feeding. She had had a double mastectomy, so couldn't breastfeed. Thus we discovered that advertising promotions for baby formula for use from birth up to six months is banned in the UK, owing to the belief they'll discourage breastfeeding.

It was a shock, as modern women, to be subjected to such paternalistic laws around what we did with our bodies and how we fed our own offspring. It felt, and it still feels, supremely patronising that mothers are not to be trusted to make their own decisions, as though we are so brainless and easily dazzled that a supermarket promotion is enough to sway us into rejecting breastfeeding outright.

Boots recently fell foul of these laws and was forced to apologise. Iceland, meanwhile, has dropped its formula prices in light of the cost of living crisis, and says it will risk an unlimited fine by advertising the fact.

In the last year, the cost of formula has shot up, but retailers are under the impression that they are not allowed to accept loyalty points, vouchers from food banks and local authorities, or store gift cards in exchange for formula. Food banks usually will not accept it either. Alongside the charity Feed and the newspaper *Metro*, Iceland has called for a change in the law. More than 40,000 people have signed a petition.

'The UK law on infant formula sale is failing; it doesn't go far enough to curtail the coercive marketing and profiteering by formula companies, but there is clear overreach in what is considered promotion, and that is penalising families,' Dr Erin Williams, co-founder and director of Feed, tells me. An urgent review is needed. 'We don't believe accepting cash equivalents as payment for infant formula is illegal, yet retailers have been led to believe this is the case. We are delighted that Iceland has taken the bold move to back our campaign and become the first UK retailer to accept cash equivalents, including loyalty points, for payment of infant formula.'

Anything written about formula usually includes the phrase 'breast is best' or some variation thereof. Iceland accepts the WHO's recommendation that babies be exclusively breastfed for the first six months. But it rightly points out that many parents, including women with medical problems, or who struggle to breastfeed, as well as gay couples and adoptive parents, simply don't have that option.

It also defends the right to choose: 'Women should be in control of their own bodies and lives, not compelled to breastfeed if they do not wish to do so,' its statement reads. 'Why in this one area should we deny them freedom? Parents are capable of making their own life choices, and should be allowed to do so.'

This made me feel like punching the air. Because breast isn't always best. I have had discussions with mental health professionals who have seen women in severe crisis because of the pressure to breastfeed. A healthy baby needs a healthy mother, but this is still not emphasised. Instead, UNICEF's controversial 'baby friendly' initiative, with its prescriptive approach, continues to influence infant feeding policy.

Of all the things I found irritating around breastfeeding culture, it was the superstitious attitude around mentioning the mere existence of formula that annoyed me the most. It was like a pre-modern belief system predicated on a spooky myth that even uttering the evil word 'formula' would jeopardise a woman's decision to do this lovely, natural thing (though, as I discovered, breastfeeding can be far from idyllic, especially at the start), like reading aloud from a book that summons demons, or standing in a dark room chanting 'Cow and Gate' in front of a mirror. Like referring to *Macbeth* as 'the Scottish play', it was cloaked in euphemism or mentioned in a kind of hushed tone.

Yet humans have historically used and needed alternatives to breastmilk. The nefarious marketing tactics of formula companies in encouraging its use, especially in the past, must of course be acknowledged (the 2023 exhibition Milk at the Wellcome Collection rightly highlighted this). But so must the fact that formula is an incredible scientific invention that saves babies' lives and helps families feed their children every single day.

Which is why some are calling for the return of National Milk, which saw formula free or subsidised by the state until 1976. Emily Baughan, a senior lecturer in history at the University of Sheffield, has written an excellent essay on its history. 'Ceasing production of National Milk in Britain never raised breastfeeding rates: that was instead the result of the increasing age and educational status of mothers,' she tells me. 'And, even now, breastfeeding rates remain low.

'The end of National Milk (and regulations on the advertisement of formula milk) has instead led to increased and unchecked profits for formula milk companies, as parents lack (and are not aware of) alternatives. Legislation intended to promote breastfeeding has had the effect of enhancing the profits of formula milk companies.

'Private companies should not be amassing major profits by providing captive, infant markets. The only way to ensure this doesn't happen is to provide a safe, NHS-endorsed and universally available alternative: to bring back National Milk.'

It's cheering to see such radical thinking around infant feeding. A thriving welfare state would also do much to encourage breastfeeding. Better funded breastfeeding support and education, a return of Sure Start, affordable access to lactation consultants, better understanding of tongue-tie and access to clinics for babies that have it, education and awareness around the benefits of combination feeding, improvements to parental leave, and perinatal mental health support – these are the things that would improve breastfeeding rates.

Until we have a government willing to prioritise these, alongside every child's right to nourishment, breastfeeding rates will remain low. But most of all, remember that fed is best. However you choose to do it.

How do you grieve for a child who barely lived? A new book has some profound answers

When Tamarin Norwood buried her son, Gabriel, the coffin was so light that it was lowered to the ground with lengths of ribbon that she had chosen herself. She writes: 'In the ribbon I saw a dull possibility: looped around his box, it would have to stay with him in the soil, and there lay some comfort. I unspooled its length into my arms and tried to kiss it all the way along, from end to end and on both sides, and pressed these handfuls of looping, folding ribbon against the wet of my eyes, held it in my arms, rocked it at my shoulder. These kisses were another last hope, sent down to his poor bones to meet them one day perhaps.'

Gabriel lived for seventy-two minutes, all spent in his mother's arms. Norwood had known that her baby boy would die. *The Song of the Whole Wide World*, her memoir of her pregnancy, his death and a maternity leave spent without a newborn, has just been published. It is a gut-wrenching tale of motherhood and loss, its sentences so pure and precise in their grief that the force of them verges on the sublime.

Norwood is not religious, yet the effect of her words feels spiritual. The book asks the question: in the absence of societal or religious rituals, how do you mourn, and mark, a life scarcely lived?

'Human beings need stories; we use stories to make sense of ourselves,' Norwood told me when we spoke. 'But when a baby dies or a pregnancy is lost, so many of the stories that we usually depend upon to make sense of death are just not there. Normally when somebody dies we are allowed to all gather together and share stories and memories about that person.'

Norwood notes that in this situation there isn't the same sense of the child having had a social place in the community: often people may not even have known you were pregnant. 'So you're all alone without those stories. You don't have those social scripts or cultural narratives of funerals and condolence cards and bereavement leave, and sometimes not even a birth and death certificate – all these things that help tell the story of the fact that somebody's died.'

'There's so much that's missing. And so what you can find is that you're going through this terrible grief, but all around you, there are no signs that you should be sad.' On top of this, family and friends often minimise the loss, saying that you can always have another one, or at least you have other children (Norwood points out that people would never say, 'You can get married again' to someone who has just lost their husband). 'And because you didn't know the baby you've lost, you don't know who you're missing. This is why grieving families often create these amazing rituals and myths in order to remember their baby. They have to write their own stories to make sense of their grief.'

Since Gabriel's death, Norwood has devoted herself to researching these mourning rituals, and working with baby-loss charities to help support parents. People often get tattoos, so a baby called 'peanut' in the womb might be remembered by the picture of a peanut on a parent's body. Butterflies and birds are frequent motifs. Special headstones in the shape of teddy bears or angels, decorated with toys and wind chimes, can be seen in cemeteries; these talismans are a sort of continuation, a need to give a lost baby the markers of a childhood that they won't see.

Siblings, too, will have their rituals. Some of the most affecting parts of Norwood's book detail how the then four-year-old Anatole, Gabriel's big brother, tries to process his death through play, acting out the ultrasound scans and later the funeral, incorporating the objects, the baby's blankets and anklets, in his memory box, and blowing kisses from his skylight towards the church where his brother has been buried.

Such scenes are unlike any I have read before, yet Anatole is not the first young sibling of an unborn or newly born baby who has had to grieve that loss. That Norwood shares these private rituals with us, where in previous years to speak of such things has been so taboo, feels like an act of supreme generosity.

Attitudes to baby loss are slowly shifting. Other writers are also exploring the issue, with the memoir *Strange Bodies* by Tom de Freston and the anthology *No One Talks About This Stuff*, edited by Kat Brown. Parents who have lost babies before twenty-four weeks of pregnancy can now apply for a certificate to mark that loss. Spending time with a baby after he or she has died, holding them, dressing them, taking casts of their hands and feet, is becoming an increasingly common practice and there are dedicated suites with refrigerated 'cuddle cots' and specialised bereavement midwives for this purpose. It is a marked shift from how previous generations were discouraged from holding or even looking at their deceased child. So many older people, Norwood says, tell her that their child was taken away before they could see them, and then scarcely spoken of again.

These days, there are charities and initiatives that can help parents in creating their rituals. Dresses for Angels makes outfits for babies 'born sleeping' (the term the charity uses) from donated wedding and bridesmaid gowns, which are given to families free of charge. Norwood has worked with Held In Our Hearts to create notelets for parents to write down their memories. Rituals can spring up organically, too. On the Parkland Walk near my house, there is a baby-loss tree with hanging ribbons and tags that bear the names of babies who have died.

There is still lots of work to do in terms of supporting bereaved families. Norwood has just embarked on a three-year project funded by the Leverhulme Trust, interviewing parents about their rituals. Her work and writing is a way of keeping her son, who 'was love itself, squirming and pushing and kicking to take up its place in the world', with her. 'To me it feels like a very small story of a very small life,' she says. 'And people are reading about it and word of mouth is spreading. You don't want a tiny life like this to just stop. It's just growing and growing.'

Afterword

I gave some thought to ending the collection with my essay on Tamarin Norwood's moving tribute to her son Gabriel, her baby who scarcely lived. I suppose I worried about readers closing the book in tears, when writing it myself made me sob on a train, or of putting a 'downer' on any of you who are expecting a child. Ultimately, though, I decided that it was important to include it for the simple reason that some people who buy this book may find themselves in similar circumstances, or know someone else who is. Those readers will still feel like parents, even though their child is no longer with them, and may be searching for some way in which to mark their loss. If the piece's inclusion contributes to a little more empathy and kindness in the world, then that will be worth the tears some of us will shed when reading about this difficult subject.

Our generation of parents are lucky in so many ways, not least in how taboos that our parents scarcely spoke of are now being let out into the open. Miscarriage, stillbirth, birth trauma, depression and loneliness used to be much harder to speak about publicly, but they are crucial aspects of parenting for many people. I write this at a time when the country's maternity services are in crisis and perinatal mental health support can be patchy and difficult to access. Admitting my own mental health struggles – and the fact that I needed support pretty much through the entire writing of this series – was difficult, but crucial if I wanted to cover the topic with honesty.

If I sometimes find myself wishing that there were more joy in parenthood writing, I still would never trade that for the secrecy and silence of the past. Years after the paediatrician and psychoanalyst David Winnicott introduced the idea of the 'good enough' mother – the reassuring concept that, while we can try to meet all our child's needs, we will sometimes fail, and that these mistakes can actually help our children learn and grow – women still face enormous pressure to be the perfect mother. This cult of perfection is such that it can make you feel like a failure to even admit that the day-to-day work of mothering isn't always sunshine and rainbows.

Reading back over these columns, particularly the early ones, one theme that emerges is how difficult parenting is when you don't have family living nearby. Since I started writing *The Republic of Parenthood,* the childcare offer in the UK has been hugely expanded, which is likely to make a very real difference to the lives of parents. Yet support isn't just about having better funding for childcare; moral support is important, too. I remain unconvinced that the nuclear family is the best environment in which to bring up children. It's not right that we are so atomised from one another; nor that we have to work so long and hard in order to cover basic housing and living costs. Yes, I do still dream of communes!

Networks that include extended family and friends (both with and without children), as well as childcare and health professionals, are a better model. Living in Islington, I feel lucky to have benefitted from something like this. Not only did the borough keep Sure Start when Tory cuts decimated the service elsewhere, but I've been pleasantly surprised by how friendly London became once I started moving around it with a baby. From women on the bus casually telling me how badly they tore in childbirth to a group of drunks in a churchyard chipping in with the chorus of 'Molly Malone' as I tried to sing him to sleep, these moments of connection felt essential.

A kind word from a stranger can turn a bad day into a good one; the other week, when I was singing to try and stave off a toddler tantrum on the bus, an older woman came up to me and said: '10/10 for what you're doing with that baby.' I could have cried. In a difficult moment, it was a vote of confidence.

I mention it not to boast, but because the differences between my generation's parenting styles and those of our parents are frequently highlighted and mocked. And there is something in that. In my writing, I try to convey how horrified my mother has been by the pressure and information overload we face. There are positives, too, of course: many of my friends who experienced quite strict and authoritarian parenting have been in therapy and are determined to be different with their own children. Our willingness to work on ourselves is, I think, something that many of today's parents can be most proud of. At the same time, there is much that we can learn from those who came before us, especially when it comes to trusting our instincts. Far from widening the generation gap, I have been pleased that my writing has gleaned a positive response from grandparents and great-grandparents as much as it has from parents my age, who feel it has helped them understand the unique challenges that their adult children are experiencing.

When you become a parent, it can be easy to feel a sudden, visceral fear and horror at the world that you have brought your baby into. Climate catastrophe, war, pandemic and political and economic instability were all global crises that coincided with the writing of this series and now book. It wasn't until I had my boy that I understood why my mum stopped watching the news after I was born. You want to exist in that blissful cocoon – in which nothing bad can ever hurt you or them, or intrude on your joy – with your baby for ever. At times it can feel as though you've been gifted pure, unadulterated happiness, alongside the terrifying fear that it could be snatched away from you in a moment. These feelings coincide in powerful ways. I have felt simultaneously a profound gratitude for my son's warmth and safety alongside an almost heartbreaking realisation that so how many children in the world do not have those privileges. There are nights where I have sat in the low nightlight red of my son's darkened bedroom and cried over the children in Gaza and the war crimes that are being committed against them.

This very raw mix of love and fear is part of what I mean when I say that parenthood can be a profoundly politicising and radicalising force. In many ways I wish it didn't have to be, that we could all exist in that blissful bubble a bit more, enjoy our babies, and worry less about external pressures and what the future has in store. Yet there is power and solidarity to be found in looking outward instead of inward, and in asking ourselves how we can work together to make the planet better for our kids.

I don't have the answers to any of these challenges, but I do know that our current model isn't working; meanwhile, politicians are panicking about the falling birth rate, and the long-term impact of an ageing population on all of us (if you're worried that not enough babies are being born, making society more hospitable to parents would be a good start). Equally, I understand that these global crises are all reasons why a person might decide not to have children; that is an entirely valid stance. As humans we are granted the ability to express love, and to give care, in myriad ways.

For those who decide to become parents, I do think that having a child in this present moment is what you might call a radical act of hope. I say this as someone who was quite anxious about becoming a mother. I worried about the intense fear that comes with the love, and about the planet, my mental health, my career, all of it. After thinking about it for a long time, and writing a book, *The Year of the Cat*, about that process, I decided to go for it. Why? Because despite all my very real concerns, I wanted to experience this all-consuming love and, in pursuing that, I couldn't help but hope for the best.

I had a high-risk pregnancy and so had to go to the hospital for monitoring fairly often. Every time I made the long shuffle to the maternity wing, I would walk past the entrance to the neonatal intensive care unit and, out of a combination of fear and superstition, I could hardly bear to look at it. I was so frightened that something would happen to my baby that to do so felt like tempting fate.

Despite my little rituals, some of those fears did come to pass: my son would, it turned out, spend some time in the NICU. It is not what I would have chosen, still isn't, but it was an important lesson in how sometimes the things that you are afraid of do actually happen, but the story never unfolds in quite the way that you imagined. It taught me that sometimes you will have to look your fear in the face before trying to move forward with renewed courage and optimism.

That's what radical hope means, I think. It's about acknowledging fears and challenges, and treating them with the respect they deserve, rather than averting our eyes. And it's also about choosing to believe that something can done to improve the state of things. I choose to find it quite inspirational that so many of us are determined to bring small beings 'into the light', as they say in Italian, and to raise them and tend to them, despite the fact that this earth can feel like a terrible, dangerous place.

Dreaming of a better world – and teaching children to do the same – feels as urgent and necessary as ever. And I do believe that there is so much that we can achieve, if we work together. If writing about my journey into motherhood has taught me anything, it's that we need one another. It's not enough to simply tread water while desperately trying to keep our heads above the waves, we have to help each other get to shore. Seeing ourselves not just within the context of our own immediate families, but as part of a larger community, has been a way of doing that for me. Throughout the writing process I've been amazed by all the people I have met who, despite often juggling their own caring responsibilities, are committed to helping others, whether it's the volunteers acting as birth companions to migrant women, or the dads campaigning for better mental health support. They are all heroes. No doubt you will meet many on your own journeys, too.

These people all share something in common, which is the belief in supporting parents as a way of caring for the babies and children they are raising. These babies will grow up to inherit the planet we all live on and most of us are united in wanting them to be a force for good in their stewardship of it. As humans we are all connected, and it is in that connection that we are offered a means of survival.

In some ways, to have a child is the least remarkable thing in the world. Billions of us have done it, stretching far back into the earliest times, and billions more will do it. Yet despite being entirely commonplace, it is also this magical, miraculous-seeming act, an act that has made me feel more profoundly linked to other women, other mothers, than ever before, as well as cementing in me an even stronger desire to prevent any child being in unnecessary pain through conflict, or cruelty, or deprivation. To feel that connection, that tenderness, and that hope so deeply and powerfully is to my mind a gift. One that must be cherished.

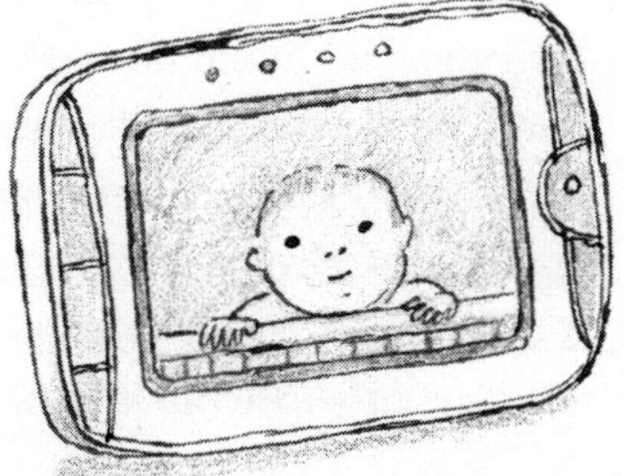

Acknowledgements

I believe all writing is a collaboration between a writer and her editor, and I could not feel more lucky to have had the support of Kirsty Major in not only dreaming up *The Republic of Parenthood* series with me, but in patiently commissioning, encouraging, steering, reshaping and, yes, cutting! Kirsty, I'm sorry that I always file too much copy and sometimes go off on tangents. You have made me a better writer. I am also eternally grateful to Jonathan Shainin, Hugh Muir, Barbara Speed, Katy Guest, Yohann Koshy, Hettie O'Brien, Lucy Pasha-Robinson and Stephen Buranyi as well as many opinion desk freelancers and of course, the production team including Rachel Aspden, Sarah Bolesworth, Phil Mongredien and Robert L. White.

I'd like to thank my agent Eleanor Birne for believing in this book, and Clare Bullock for her vision and creativity in making it. It's even more beautiful than I ever could have imagined. Everyone at September Publishing has been so enthusiastic and supportive – thank you so much to all of you, as well as to Tabitha Pelly, for championing it. And Pia: you are a true artist and I am so, so lucky have worked with you on this.

To all the people who spoke to me, patiently allowing me to interview them while my baby whinged in the background or wriggled at the breast: thank you. Many of you shared intensely personal, sometimes difficult things with me and I hope that I have honoured those experiences. And to the readers of the column, so many of whom have thoughtfully emailed, messaged, and commented – you make it all worthwhile.

Both raising a baby and writing a book take a village and I couldn't have done any of it without the army of professionals who have supported us throughout, from the maternity and paediatric staff at the Whittington hospital to health visitors Kerry and Stephanie, breastfeeding counsellor Karen, and lactation consultant Sue Freeman. Special thanks to Dr Catrin Cooper, as well as the perinatal mental health team, especially Pendra, whose visits in the early days meant the world. Thank yous are not enough.

Marta – I said I was going to send you a thank-you card but I was waiting until I felt I was able to tell you that I was OK, and then I never did. So this is my belated thank you: I am OK, and it is largely because of you. Thank you for rewiring my brain in ways that I cannot begin to articulate, for your insight and intelligence, and for saying things like: 'Please forgive me for being a bit Lacanian for a moment.' That I got to work with you for free on the NHS remains astonishing to me.

To the women in the baby and toddler rooms who have cared for my son, who have held him and rocked him and cuddled him and fed him and comforted him, and who have taught him so many things: I owe you a great debt. Particular thanks to Cristina, Ewa, Fatima, Fittoria, Lufta, Marie, Rose, Shadia, Sumayyah, Tahiya, Sophie and, of course, the wonderful Zuzana.

Special thanks to 'Archway Mamas' Liza, Jess and Sian – I think I'd have drowned in the warm soup of motherhood without your humour, camaraderie, and support. The same is true of Jane, Holly and Theresa; I'm so glad I met you. I'm also eternally grateful to Anna Steadman, the *capo* of the 'Mat leave Mondays' group and rhyme time socialite extraordinaire. Gav: I get the sense that you're uncomfortable with public displays of emotion, so I'll just say 'Ta' and get you a pint.

Thanks to Bryony, Leja and Hazel for continuing to make me howl with laughter. To Holly: despite the ocean between us, I somehow feel that you have been by my side throughout our journeys in early motherhood. You're a true comrade. And to Shakes, Sarah, Nats, Katherine, Louise, Emily, Sian, Lucia, Olive, Rebecca, Elizabeth for your friendship and support.

I owe special thanks to Jessica. Your voicenotes, your kindness, your wisdom, and your solidarity have meant the world.

To fake siblings Kim, Hannah and, of course, to Kate. How privileged I am to have shared a childhood with the three of you. Kate, I still can't believe you are gone – though your smile lives on in AK. I will never forget your reaction when I told you my news. I know the thought that Hannah and I would become mums together gave you some comfort, and I hope it still does wherever you are (in my mind, you are soaring above the Himalayas).

Most of all, I am grateful to our families. I'm especially thankful to Emily, Theresa, Clare, and Jane (Jane, I'm so sorry I sent you pictures of shitty nappies when you were probably trying to have lunch. I jest, but you and your medical knowledge may have saved my baby's life or prevented him from becoming very poorly on at least one occasion. Thank you.)

To Rob and Diana, and all of the sibs, spouses and cousins. Thank you for the love you have shown our boy. Diana, I still can't believe you have birthed and raised nine children. You have been a wonderful sounding board, and somehow despite your vast experience in motherhood have never made me feel like an amateur.

Siâni, *diolch o galon am bopeth. Cariad mawr mawr.*

To Mum and Dad: without you, I would not have got through this. Mum: I'm so sorry that you spent so many nights on our sofa. I still feel guilty about it. What a joy and an honour, though, to have you there with me. And Dad, seeing you become a Taid has been so wonderful. Words will never be enough for either of you: thank you.

I owe the greatest debt to Tim, for being the most wonderful husband and dad to our little Bug. You've put in a shift, to say the least. How lucky I am to get to do this with you. We love you so much.

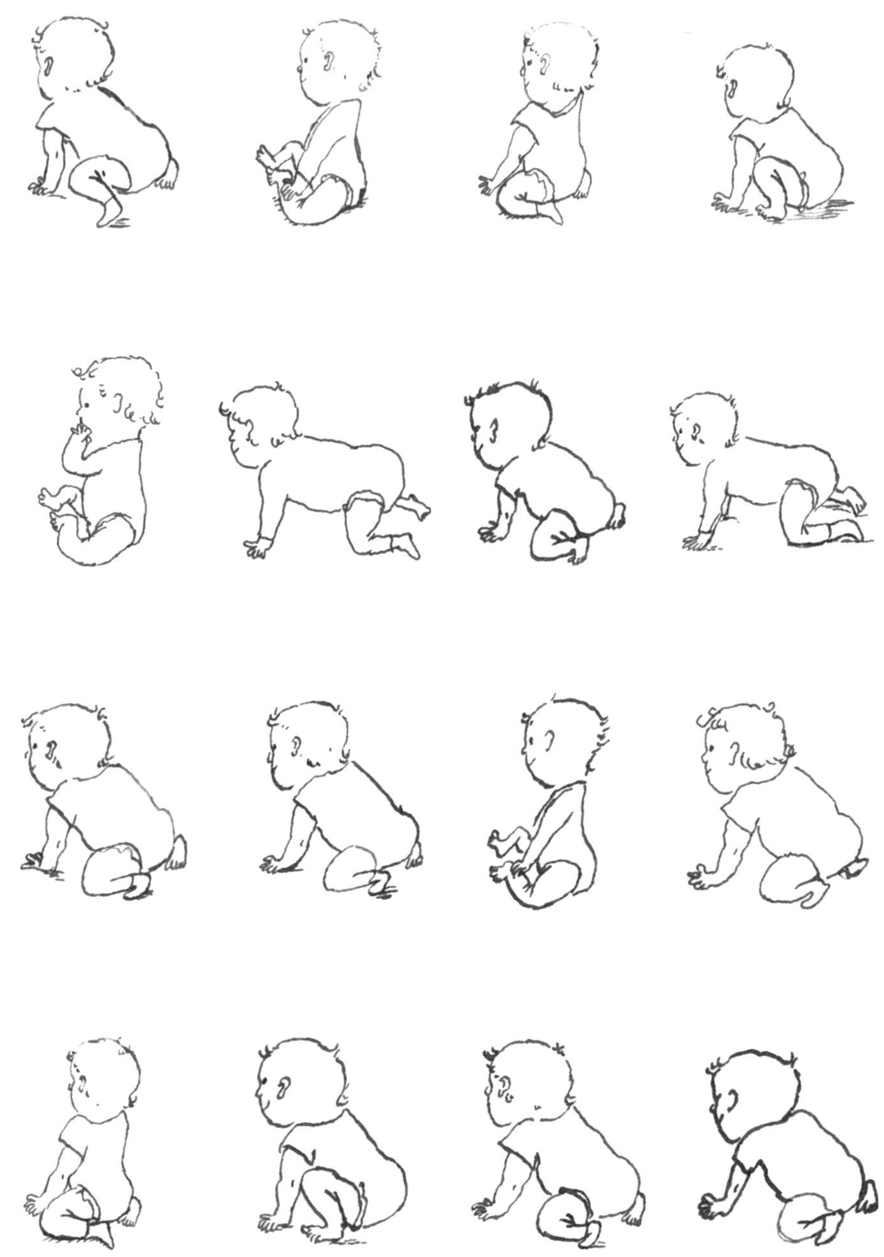